Natural Vibrant Health
Raw Food

Kendell Reichhart, Holistic Health Counselor & Nutritional Consultant
Brian Hetrich, Certified Nutritional Counselor

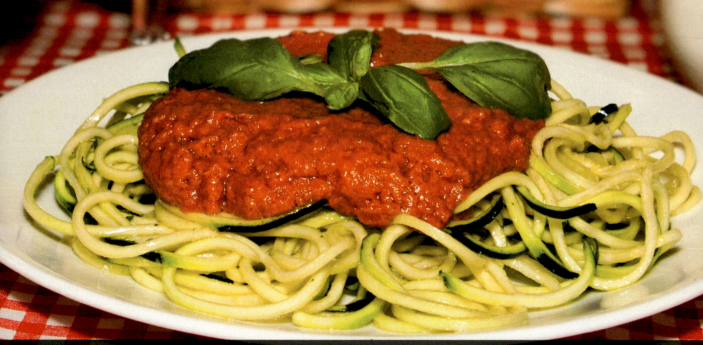

A Brian Hetrich, LLC Publication

RECIPES FOR LIVING

Publisher
Brian Hetrich, LLC

Photograghy
JAX Audio/Video, LLC
http://www.JaxAudioVideo.Com

Cover Art, Design, Layout & Editing
Living Food Network, LLC
http://www.LivingFoodNetwork.Org

For More Information Contact:
Natural Vibrant Health
31 Allegheny Avenue, Suite 202
Towson, Maryland 21204
(443) 250-9335
http://www.NaturalVibrantHealth.Net

Copyright © 2011 Brian Hetrich, LLC
All rights reserved. This book may not be reproduced in whole or in part without written permission from the publisher, except by a reviewer who may quote brief passages in a review, nor may any part of this book be reproduced, stored in a retrieval system, or transmitted in any form or by any means, electronic, mechanical, photocopying, recording, or other, without written permissions from Brian Hetrich, LLC.

ISBN-10: 1461187206
ISBN-13: 978-1461187202

Medical Disclaimer:

The food, food preparation and health information in this book is based on the training, experience and research of the authors and is intended to inform and educate. Check with a qualified health professional prior to beginning this or any health program. The author and publisher specifically disclaim any liability, loss, or risk, personal or otherwise, which is incurred as a consequenece, directly or indirectly, of the use and application of the contents of this book.

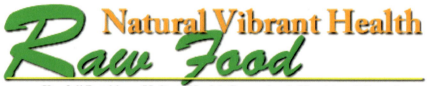

Acknowledgements

I would like to thank the person who introduced me to raw foods, Dr. Jim Sharps. His example, wise counsel, and motivation inspired and cast me off on an absolutely amazing health journey that has completely turned my life around for the better. I have learned that nothing tastes as good as good health feels. Thanks, Dr. Sharps!

- Brian

I would like to acknowledge the raw food guru, David Wolfe. As I started making the changes in my life and diet, I met David Wolfe, an amazing speaker and author who travels the world lecturing on Natural Health, Nutrition, and Healing. I went on one of his raw retreats in Sedona, Arizona, and really learned how to heal the body at a cellular level through proper nutrition, and amazing foods and herbs. He has been an inspiration to me along my health journey. Thanks, Avocado!

- Kendell

RECIPES FOR LIVING

Table of Contents

Acknowledgements	3
Forward	6
About the Authors	7
Kendall Reichart	8
Credentials	9
Brian Hetrich	10
Why We Wrote This Book	12
Why Raw Foods?	13
Kitchen Tools	15
High-Speed Blender	15
Food Processor	16
Dehydrator	16
Juicer	17
Spiralizer	18
Nut Milk Bag	18
Sprouting Jars	18
Julienne Slicer	19
Mandolin	19
About Ingredients	20
Raw	20
Fresh	20
Ripe	20
Organic	21
Local	22
Plant-based	22
Standardized Measurements	23
Smoothies	25
Kendall's Green Smoothie	26
Super-Power Smoothie	27
Cherry-Fire Smoothie	28
Memory Nut Nog	29
Blueberry Basil Smoothie	31
Very Berry Smoothie	32
Blue Smoothie	33
Fruit Chard Smoothie	34
Mocha Chocolate Milkshake	35
Ultimate Smoothie	36
Maca Blast	37
Peachy Green Smoothie	38
Kale Smoothie	39
Drinks & Juices	41
Almond Milk	42
Blood Builder	43
Green Machine	44
Kombucha	45
Great Awakenings	46
Super Nova Sun Tea	47
Soups	49
Veggie Miso Soup	50
Noodles	50
Soup Base	50
Garnish	50
Spinach Curry	51
Italian Wedding Soup	52
Garnish	52
Winter Squash Soup	53
Sweet Potato Soup	54
Mushroom Soup	55
Soup Base	55
Soup Topping	55
Thai Soup	56
Fiesta Soup	57
Salads	59
What About Vitamin D?	60
Kale Salad	61
Cauliflower Sprout Salad	62
Salad	62
Dressing	62
Garnish	62
Entrees & Sides	63
Protein	65
Raw Burritos	66
Cashew Sour Cream	66
Guacamole	66
Taco Meat	66
Stuffed Bell Peppers	67
Cauliflower Rice	68
Raw Lasagna	69
Noodles	69
Pesto	69
Marinara	69
Ricotta	69
Cheezy Cauliflower Casserole	70
"Cheeze" Topping	70
Pad Thai	71
Sauce	71
Noodles	71
Toppings	71
Tuna Wraps	72
Pizza	74
Bread	74
Tomato Sauce	75
Cheese	75
Chili	76
Garnish	76
Dolmas	77
Spaghetti	78
Pasta	78
Marinara	78
Sweet Potato Casserole	79
Topping	79
Burgers	81
Paté	81
Buns	81
Raw Ketchup	81
Spicy Jicama Fries	82
Savory Jicama Fries	83
Tabouli	84
Snacks	85
Flax Crackers	86
Ricotta Cheese	87
Famous Flax Crackers	88
Zucchini Hummus	89
Guacamole	90
Walnut Hummus	91
Spicy Nacho Kale Chips	92
Desserts	93
Cacao Power Balls	94
Chocolate Macaroons	94
Chocolate Brownies	95
Brownie	95
Icing	95
Apple Pie	96
Crust	96
Filling	96
Topping	96
Drizzle Garnish	96
Blueberry Cheesecake	97
Crust	97
Filling	97
Topping	97
Key Lime Pie	98
Crust	98
Filling Ingredients	98
Peach Pecan Cobbler	99
Pumpkin Pie	100
Strawberry Crepes	101
Ice Cream	102
Chocolate Moose	103
Raw Food Studies	104
Food Glossary	107
Index	115

4 - *Raw Food* – NATURAL VIBRANT HEALTH

NATURAL VIBRANT HEALTH – RAW FOOD

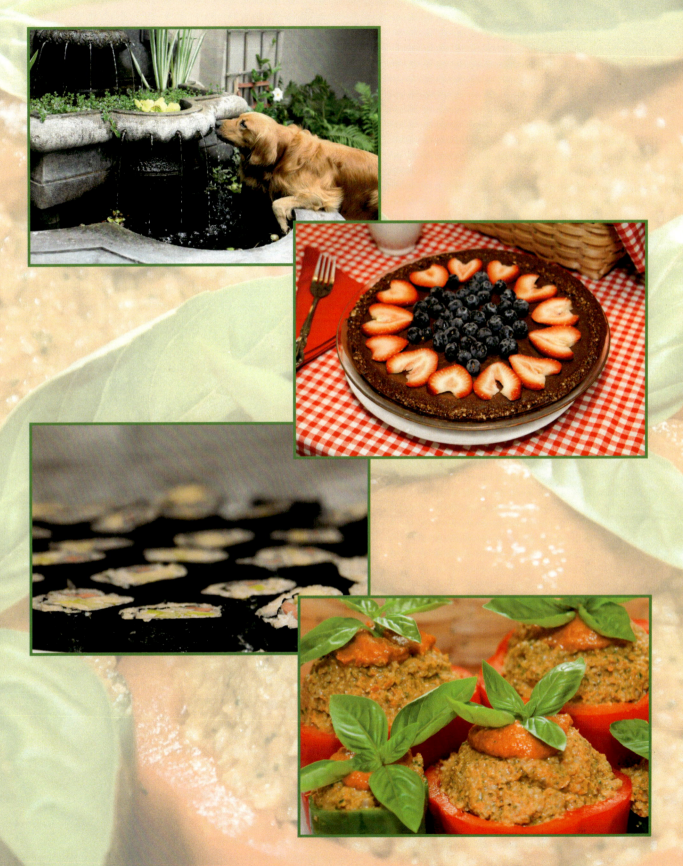

RECIPES FOR LIVING – *Raw Food* - 5

RECIPES FOR LIVING

Forward

I love raw food! The maximum quality and quantity of nutrients in raw food helps to keep my coat shiny. The enzymes in raw food are the catalyst for every chemical reaction in my body which gives me energy for the important things in life. Like,

- **Chasing the ball**
- **Chasing squirrels**
- **Chasing rabbits**
- **Running away with someone's flip-flops**

I also love going to work with Kendell. Sometimes, I get to stop by Zia's for some raw crackers for lunch or walking to and from the office. I serve as the official taste tester at the Clean Water Class and I always choose the spring water over the tap water. I even get to sample some of the leftovers from the raw food "cooking" classes which use recipes from this book. I just want you all to know that I heartedly endorse this book.

— Jake

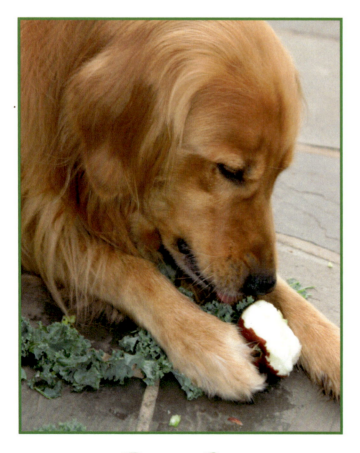

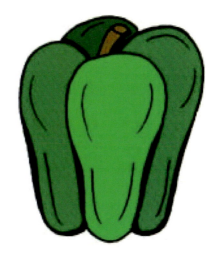

"About the Authors"

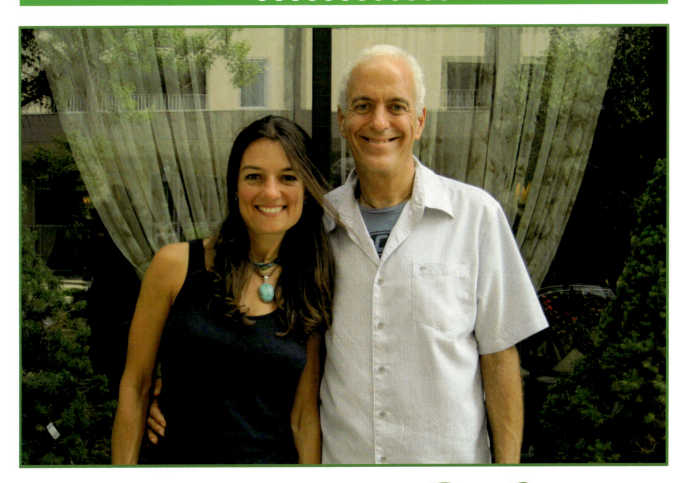

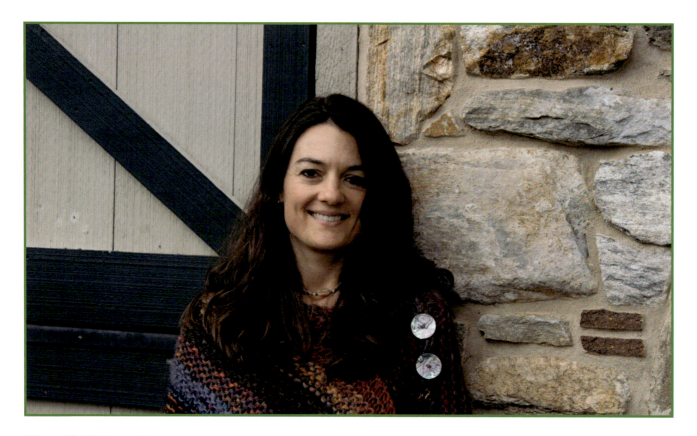

Kendell Reichart

I have been intrigued with the field of nutrition since I was a child. I read the labels on everything, even at the age of seven. I saw that calories meant energy, so I ate more calories so that I would have more energy. Those labels do not mean the same anymore.

What brought me into the world of Holistic Health was the battles with my own health. I grew up with a lot of digestive issues and fatigue. After college, I was professionally competing and training horses, but was always exhausted with severe stomach and digestive disorders and debilitating menstrual issues. I was constantly at the doctor, even at a young age, and usually getting the same answers..."your fine". I sure didn't feel fine!! Eventually I was told I had Chronic Fatigue Syndrome, depression and anxiety. I started having breathing issues, which they told me was the anxiety. I wanted to know "WHY" I had these problems and felt this way, but would never get an answer, just a prescription... This led me to started doing my own research and seek out alternative means of health and healing. From here I learned about adrenal fatigue and started to understand what was really going on inside my body. I researched stomach and digestive issues and started weeding out certain foods. Next, I got some food allergy testing done with a naturopath, discovered I was highly allergic to eggs and this was the cause of my breathing issues! Then found out I COULD NOT eat gluten (Celiac's Disease), which was the root cause of most of my health issues. Many years of trying to figure out my own problems, and healing them naturally mostly through diet and some amazing supplements and herbs, led me to where I am now. With the knowledge I gained by healing from the inside out, I knew I needed to help others learn to do the same.

As I started making the changes in my life and diet, I met David Wolfe, an amazing speaker and author who travels the world lecturing on Natural Health, Nutrition, and Healing. I went on one of his raw retreats in Sedona Arizona, and really learned how to heal the body at a cellular level through proper nutrition, and amazing foods and herbs. What I have learned over the past few years on this path has been amazing, and the level of energy that I have now achieved is better than I can ever remember since I was a child. My outlook on life has been completely renewed and now I do everything I can to share this knowledge and information, and help others obtain the same goals of optimum health!

Professional Credentials

Kendell Reichhart is a Holistic Health Counselor and Nutritional Consultant was associated with the Cometa Wellness Center in Lutherville, MD before opening her own practice in Towson October 1st, 2009. Kendell completed her undergraduate studies at the University of Maryland, where she received a B.S. in Biology and Psychology. She received her nutritional education in the Professional Training Program of the Institute for Integrative Nutrition. Through this program, Kendell received certification and accreditation from The Center for Educational Outreach and Innovation of the Teachers College at Columbia University, and from the American Association of Drugless Practitioners. She has continued her education by completing a workshop in Raw Foods and Healing Herbs at the Omega Institute for Holistic Studies.

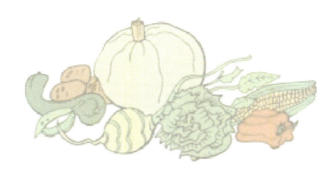

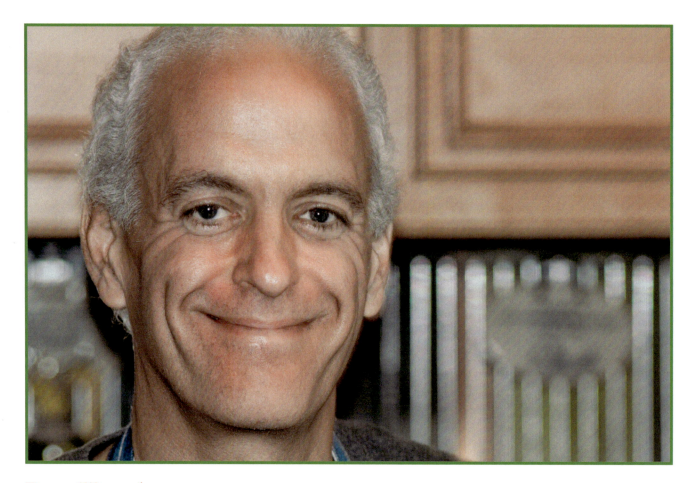

Brian Hetrich

I lived most of my life eating the Standard American Diet (SAD.) My health suffered as a result and I became seriously overweight, tired all the time and developed a whole host of chronic ailments including headaches, backaches, high blood pressure, high cholesterol, it seemed like I was sick all the time, low energy, allergies, acne, poor vision, brain fog, poor sleep to name a few. I reluctantly accepted this as normal because the same thing seemed to be happening to almost everybody else. Finally, I became just plain sick and tired of being sick and tired. I tried every diet and every kind of exercise I could think of, and nothing worked. I began searching for a change.

In January 2005 I attended a lecture on health given by a very fit-looking naturopath, Dr. Jim Sharps. He claimed that going on a "raw food diet" was the most amazing thing he had ever done in his life. I found his presentation compelling and inspirational. I decided to make some small changes to my meals and began to move towards a more plant-based diet. I went vegetarian for a year then, vegan for a year and then "high raw" for a year. Every step of the way I noticed more and more improvements to my health. I was very intrigued by these positive changes and decided to go 100% raw just to see what would happen.

I simply cannot overemphasize the amazing power of raw foods! To say that going from SAD to 100% raw is like "night and day" is an understatement. It is more like being transformed to another dimension! Not only did I quickly lose 100 pounds of excess weight and all of my health challenges go away but, my mental clarity, focus, awareness, sensitivity and sense of connectedness soared to levels I never knew existed! Without me realizing it this new found sense of awareness and energy began to steer my life in another direction. After spending 25 years in the corporate world, I decided to make a career change.

I enrolled in the Doctor of Naturopathy in Original Medicine degree program at the International Institute of Original Medicine. In September of 2010, I left my job at Honeywell to launch a new career in the field of nutritional health. I teamed up with Kendell to offer some of the latest, most cutting-edge information on health and wellness to the Baltimore area. Our goal is to give people the best possible resources so they can make the most educated choices to improve their health and optimize wellness. Together, we have been conducting regularly scheduled raw food cooking classes, potlucks, raw chocolate parties, movie nights and health education lectures. I also counsel individuals on nutrition with a focus on healthy meal planning and weight management.

The nutritional constituents listed in this book for each food item and their corresponding beneficial value to the human body is not meant to be a comprehensive list. We have listed just one of the predominant nutritional components and just one of its corresponding benefits in order to keep this book succinct. For example, magnesium is just one of dozens of the nutritional constituents found in Swiss chard and it is used in over 300 chemical processes in the body. Nutritional scientists are learning about more nutritional components found in food and their uses by the human body every day.

Why We Wrote This Book

We both came from a place of many years of less than vibrant health. We were searching for a solution. We discovered the answer at about the same time but, in different places. The irony is that that answer is so simple and it is literally right at our feet! The key to vibrant health is in whole, living foods in their purest, most natural state. The further you stray from nature the less healthy you will be. When we realized this fact and experienced an amazing transformation in our own lives we could not help but get excited and have the desire to share this incredible information with others. We started conducting raw food prep classes to demonstrate methods of preparing "gourmet" dishes that taste great and are very healthy for you. This book contains recipes we have been teaching in those classes.

Your body is incredible! It has self-healing mechanisms built right in. When you change your diet for the better you will experience a corresponding improvement in your health and well being. There is a direct correlation between the degree to which you improve your diet and how good you will feel. While there are many diets that are an improvement on the Standard American Diet (SAD) we are convinced that the best way to eat is whole, living foods in their purest, most natural state. The big news is not that fruits and vegetables are good for you. The big news is that fruits and vegetables are so good for you that they can totally change you, turn your life around and save your life! Remember, nothing tastes as good as good health feels!

One of our favorite quotes is, "When health is absent, wisdom cannot reveal itself, art cannot manifest, strength is not to be found, wealth becomes useless, and reason becomes powerless." - Herophiles, 300 B.C., Physician to Alexander the Great. Raw food and the corresponding vibrant health that comes along with it is a means to an end. We are all incredible beings and we all have an important mission to fulfill on this planet. When you have vibrant health it becomes possible for you to fulfill that mission. When you do not have your health every endeavor that you attempt becomes difficult. We both have a passion for nature and the planet. We want to save the world. We intend to do just that. Why don't you join us?

Why Raw Foods?

No other creature in the wild on this planet cooks their food before eating it. Except humans. And, no other creature in the wild suffers the debilitating illnesses such as cancer, diabetes, heart disease, arthritis, osteoporosis except humans. You were born into this world with everything you need to survive and thrive. You were not born into this world with a stove or microwave attached to your belly. Cooking denatures food. The life-giving and healing nutrients available in food are heat sensitive. On average, the cooking process destroys at least 50% of the minerals and fiber, 75% of the protein and vitamins and 100% of the hormones, oxygen, phytonutrients and enzymes in food. Cooking also renders food toxic by creating free radicals through a process call glycation.

Enzymes are large protein molecules found in all living things – plant and animal. Your body is capable of producing two types of enzymes, metabolic and digestive. In human physiological terms, metabolic enzymes are the spark of life. They are the catalyst for every single chemical reaction in your body - every process, every action, every muscle movement, every sense, every thought, every word and every deed. The more enzymes you have inside of you the more alive you become. Food in its' original, fresh, ripe, raw and unadulterated state contains naturally occurring enzymes which aid in its' own digestion. When a peach falls to the ground the cell walls are broken and a bruise develops at the point of contact. The enzymes are liberated and the peach begins to digest itself. The same process occurs when we chew the peach. This greatly reduces the burden of digestion from your body since it does not have to go through the taxing process of manufacturing enzymes for the digestion of the peach.

This is a key point as the body expends a great deal of energy in the digestion of food. When you eat a cooked food meal, 80% of your body's total available energy is expended in the processing of that meal. When you eat a raw food meal the energy expended in processing is reduced to only 20%. The less energy you expend on digestion the more energy you have available for life. Most people go through their entire lives totally unaware of their true potential because their bodies are perpetually under the heavy burden of processing the unnatural foods they are eating. The more food is processed the more enzymes are destroyed and it becomes mostly "dead." Because of their highly perishable nature, heat processing (cooking) destroys 100% of the enzymes in foods rendering it completely inert. This increases shelf life which is very desirable for the commercial food distribution industry but, it is highly undesirable for your body's health and well-being.

RECIPES FOR LIVING

As a result of cooking and other forms of food processing, enzymes are largely missing from the Standard American Diet (SAD.) Other essential nutrients such as vitamins, minerals and proteins are also destroyed in the processing of food which creates other issues with your health. Your body has the capability of producing digestive enzymes to make up for the lack of enzymes in cooked and otherwise processed foods. The problem is that you were born with a finite ability to manufacture enzymes. When you deplete your enzyme manufacturing capability, you die. The less of a burden you put on your body to produce digestive enzymes, the more metabolic enzymes will be available throughout your lifespan. This greatly improves your energy, vitality, health and longevity. This is part of the magic and life force energy in raw foods. Raw foods are alive and we are alive. Life begets life. Hence, the more raw living foods you eat the more alive you become! It is not uncommon to see people who eat mostly raw foods to look 15 years younger than their true chronological age and have soaring energy levels. Raw foods are truly anti-aging! Living foods create living bodies in vibrant health. Cooked food is dead which create sick, decaying and dead bodies.

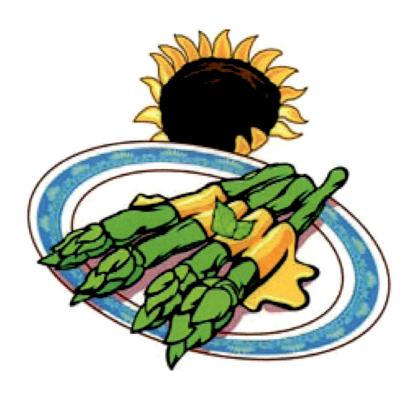

Kitchen Tools

Every well-stocked kitchen contains tools and appliances for preparing meals. Things like sharp knives, cutting boards, peelers, measuring spoons and cups, coffee grinders, stoves, ovens, toasters, and microwaves are common in most kitchens. Some of these tools are shared in a raw food kitchen. However, we frequently use tools that are typically not found in a cooked food kitchen - some of which may be unfamiliar to you. Things like high speed blenders, food processors, dehydrators, juicers, sprouting jars, and spiralizers are used for some of the recipes in this book. You may already own some of these appliances but, they are infrequently used. If you are unfamiliar with how to use these appliances you may find it helpful to attend a raw food prep class in your area for instruction.

If you do not already own all of these specialized raw food tools, acquiring them may seem like a bit of a hurdle. We can unequivocally assure you that the initial investment is well worth the health dividends you will reap for years to come! Good health comes through the kitchen, not through the medicine cabinet. Think of all the money you are going to save on doctor visits, prescription co-pays, missed sick days, etc. Also, your utility bill will go down because you are not cooking, baking, frying, toasting, microwaving, or grilling. Not to mention you never have to worry about burning or over cooking! In some cases you can substitute one tool or method for another.

High-Speed Blender

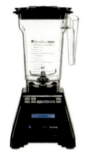

This is the most frequently used appliance in our kitchen. It liquefies ingredients and is therefore useful for making smoothies, soups, sauces, dressings, nut butters, nut milks, ice cream and more. The high-speed blender works just like a standard blender but with greater capacity, higher speed blades, and a more powerful motor. These features are very helpful for working with raw plant-based ingredients that are high in fiber and cellulose. The motor on a high-speed blender is much larger and stronger than a standard blender. The blades in a high-speed blender rotate up to 23,000 revolutions per minute which is about 20 times faster than a standard blender. This high speed helps to shred and open up the cell walls of the tough plants making the nutrients in them more easily accessible and available to our body's cells. If you leave it run a little longer, this feature also is useful for gently warming foods (like soups) due to the friction created by the high speed blades. It technique only takes a minute or two and you just want to bring the food up to about body temperature.

RECIPES FOR LIVING

There are several good high-speed blenders on the market. Two excellent brands are Vitamix and Blendtec. The Vitamix comes with a plunger (tamper) while the Blendtec uses a "vortex" action to process heavy mixes. The Vitamix is available with a variable speed knob while the Blentec features digital controls with some pre-programmed keys. Because of its' versatility and usefulness, this is the first appliance you should consider adding to your kitchen.

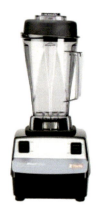

You can use a standard blender for most applications in place of the high-speed blender. However, it will take longer and you will need to pre-chop things up by hand into smaller chunks prior to placing in the blender. You should avoid attempting certain recipes in a standard blender such as nut butters, ice cream and dehydrated tomatoes as this will burn up the motor. You can also substitute a food processor for most recipes in place of the high-speed blender. But, the food processor has a much lower liquid limit capacity and therefore, is not as useful for things like smoothies and nut milks. In general, the high-speed blender is the best tool for high liquid content mixes.

Food Processor

The function of the food processor is similar to that of the high-speed blender except that the latter liquefies ingredients while the former is primarily designed to chop food into smaller pieces. However, if you leave the food in the food processor long enough you will almost get the consistency that you would in a blender. It is a versatile tool and comes with several different blades. The "S" blade is used for blending and chopping. We use it often for making pizza crust and pie crusts from nuts and dates. The shredding

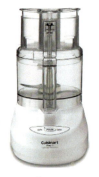

blade is used for making small chards of food from cabbage for things like sauerkraut and cole slaw. In lieu of using the food processor with the shredding blade you can use a hand shredder if you have the time. The slicing blade is used for making thin slices of food for things like apples slices for apple pie. In lieu of the slicing blade you can use a knife and cutting board. Obviously, the food processor would be a lot quicker. There are many good food processors on the market. We like the larger, 14-cup models.

Dehydrator

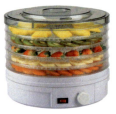

The dehydrator is basically a low-temperature convection oven. A standard oven contains only heaters. A convection oven con-

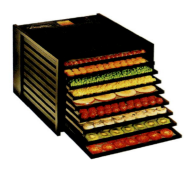
tains heaters and fans to move the air over the food to speed the drying process. Dehydrating draws the water out of food without cooking it. This process concentrates the flavor in food and helps to preserve it. Adding a dehydrator to your kitchen repertoire really helps you to make the transition from the SAD to raw lifestyle a little easier. It allows you to make "fun foods" like flax, crackers, corn chips, pizza crust, and kale chips. These foods help to satiate those cravings for starchy carbohydrates in a healthy way. You can also use the dehydrator to warm your raw food soups and other dishes up to body temperature which can be more pleasing in the colder months.

Once again, there are many different models of dehydrators on the market. Make sure you get one with an adjustable thermostat that will allow you to set the temperature at 105 degrees F. by keeping the temperature below 105 degrees F you preserve most of the precious heat-sensitive nutrients like enzymes that are absent in cooked food. We like the square-tray models which allow you to make pizza crusts.

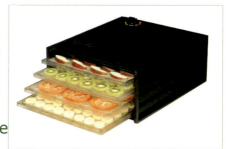

Juicer

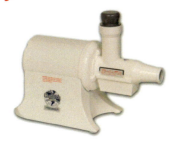
A juicer extracts the liquids from fruits and vegetables and separates it from the indigestible fiber and pulp. The juice is the blood of the plants. Juicing opens up the cell walls of the tough plants making the nutrients in them more easily accessible and available to our body's cells. For example, you only absorb 2% of the beta carotene when you eat a carrot. However, when you juice a carrot you absorb 100% of the beta carotene! The Champion is a high speed shredding juicer while the Omega VRT, GreenStar and GreenPower are slow speed compression juicers. These all do a great job for fruits, vegetables and dark leafy greens including wheatgrass (a special leafy-green attachment is needed for the Champion.) We sometimes use a hand-crank juicer for wheatgrass. We also sometimes use a separate citrus juicer for oranges, lemons, limes and grapefruit.

In lieu of a juicer you can make juice by first liquefying the food using a blender or food processor and then straining the slurry through a nut milk bag.

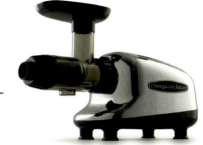

RECIPES FOR LIVING

Spiralizer

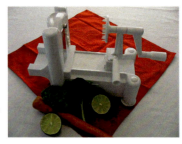

This relatively inexpensive tool is another favorite in our kitchen! This easy-to-use and fun accoutrement quickly makes noodles and pasta shapes out of zucchini or other vegetables and hard fruits. Unlike the shredder blade in the food processor or a hand shredder, the Spiralizer makes long, continuous strands of veggie noodles or pasta. This device is ideal for making the zucchini noodles used in our spaghetti recipe. Different blades are included with most models for making different shapes and sizes of veggie noodles and pasta.

Nut Milk Bag

A nut milk bag is used for straining the liquid from the pulp of slurries made in the blender or food processor. It is idea for making almond milk for which it is most often used. Simply pour the slurry mix into the nut milk bag while holding it over a large bowl. Bring in the drawstring and massage the nut milk bag to squeeze all the moisture out of the slurry. Save the pulp for bread recipes in the dehydrator.

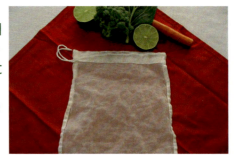

You can also grow sprouts in a nut milk bag. Simply place the sprout seeds in the nut milk bag and soak in a pan of water for the recommended period of time based on the type of sprouts. Then, lift the bag out of the water to drain and, using the drawstring, suspend the bag over a pan. Immerse the bag in water twice a day and immediately hang back up until the sprouts are done.

Sprouting Jars

This is nothing more than one-quart wide mouth Mason jars with special sprouting lids. The sprouting lids have screened tops instead of the closed tops on the normal lids. These lids can be purchased separately at any hard-core health food store. Simply place the sprout seeds in the Mason jars, screw on the sprouting lid, fill with water and soak for the recommended period of time based on the type of sprouts. Then, turn the jar upside down in the sink to drain and leave in this position in the sink or at a 45 degree angle in a dish rack. Rinse the sprout seeds twice a day and immediately drain and leave upside down until the sprouts are done. We prefer jars made in the USA because there is less chance that they contain heavy metals and other toxins potentially found in glass sourced from some foreign countries.

Julienne Slicer

This hand-held tool uses a two-stage blade system to create matchstick-sized string cuts from vegetables and hard fruits. The results are similar to using the shredding blade in the food processor only finer. Be sure to use the food guard and watch those blades!

Mandolin

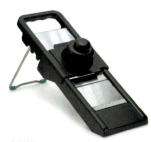

A mandolin allows you to make straight, thin slices from vegetables and hard fruits. This instrument has a height adjustment to allow you to vary the thickness of the product. It is similar to using the slicing blade in the food processor only you can get thinner slices. This is the tool of choice for the zucchini noodles in our raw lasagna recipe. Again, please be sure to use the food guard and watch those blades!

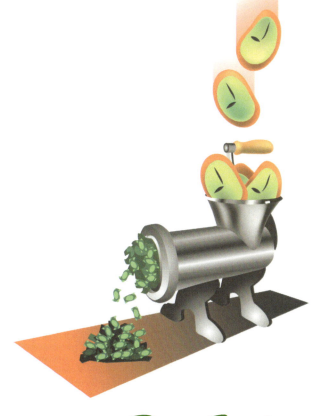

RECIPES FOR LIVING

A Few Words About Ingredients

All of your ingredients should be sourced as raw, fresh, ripe, organic, whole, local, and plant-based. While discussing the importance of each one of these characteristics warrants it's own book, we will highlight just a few of the highlights here for the sake of brevity. It is best if you plant a garden in your backyard and grow as much of your own food as possible. This allows you to better control the quality of your food.

Raw

This is the most important characteristic for all your ingredients. Nothing used in your recipes should ever have been heated by any process above 105 degrees F. Temperatures above this point destroy the majority of the nutrients, energy, enzymes and life force in food. Furthermore, cooking food chemically alters certain food components and renders it toxic. In general, your grocery shopping should be limited to the fresh produce section of the store. You should buy only food that resembles the condition as it appears in nature. Most things that come in a box, jar, can, bottle or bag have been cooked, pasteurized or heat processed in some way and should be avoided. The exceptions are those things that are specifically labeled "raw", "cold-pressed", "sun-dried", "unpasteurized" or "not heated over 105 degrees F".

Fresh

The sooner you consume your food to harvest time the better. Even when food is not heated it quickly begins to lose some of its' nutritional value and flavor as soon as it is harvested. The best way to achieve freshness is to grow your own at home. The next best option is to buy as much produce as you can from your local farmer's market or roadside stand that carries local produce. The sight, smell, touch, taste, and sound of food will be best at its' peak of freshness. Use your five senses to evaluate your food for freshness before you buy it. Ask the produce manager when the food was harvested and when it was delivered. Patronize those stores that sell the freshest produce. Only buy enough food for a couple of days supply. This means you will shop more often and buy less food on each trip. Use fresh herbs and spices as much as possible. The flavor and nutritional value of fresh herbs and spices is much better compared to the dried versions sold in a bottle, can, jar, bag or box.

Ripe

The taste and nutritional value of food is also at its' peak when it is allowed to ripen on the vine, tree or bush before harvesting. This gives the plant the time it needs to absorb the maximum amount of nutrients from the soil, air, rain, and sunshine. You can tell when some produce like apples, peaches, pears, tomatoes, etc. are ripe because they will fall to the earth on its' own when you shake it. Certain foods that are harvested before they are allowed to ripen are too acidic and drain minerals from the body. Unfortunately, commercially distributed fruit is always picked many weeks before it is ripe. This is done because it extends the shelf life of the product at the expense of flavor and nutritional value. Whenever possible, you should grow your own food or buy your produce locally from a farmer's market that does not pick their produce before it is ripe.

Organic

Conventional produce is sprayed heavily with chemical pesticides, herbicides, and fungicides that are extremely harmful to your body. Some of these dangerous chemicals penetrate deeply into the flesh of the produce and cannot be washed off. Also, some non-organic food is irradiated which stops the division of life, thereby killing the food. Artificial chemical fertilizers used on conventional produce accelerate the plant growth which does not allow the plants to develop naturally and extract all the nutrients that it would. Conventional produce is usually devoid of most essential minerals because artificial chemical fertilizers contain only nitrogen, potassium, and phosphorus. The other 89 minerals are missing[1]. Some conventional food is now genetically modified (GMO) to increase profits. Genetically modified means scientists are injecting the DNA from one plant into the DNA of a totally different plant or even between different species such as between animals and plants to create new "frankenfoods." There have not been enough long-term tests to understand the full impact of such genetic manipulation. There is no requirement for GMO labeling in the USA. It is estimated that upwards of 70 percent of all processed foods on supermarket shelves in the USA now contain genetically engineered ingredients[2]. We believe that you should not put anything GMO in your body. GMO foods should be avoided at all costs. In most countries, organic products do not contain GMOs.

Whole

The nutrient loss in food is accelerated as soon as it is cut, peeled, chopped, mashed, heated, or processed in any way. Ideally, the first thing that cuts into your food should be your teeth. The next best thing is for you to obtain your food whole and prepare it at home just moments before you eat it.

---

[1] Charlotte Gerson, "Food Matters"
[2] The True Food Network, Center for Food Safety

Local

Most commercially distributed produce in the USA is picked up to two weeks prior to showing up for sale on store shelves. This does not account for produce imported from outside our borders. In that case the number of days between picking and delivery and the miles travelled increase dramatically which has a huge impact on the potential freshness and the potential ripeness of your food. Most food that is shipped great distances is grown on large factory farms using unsustainable practices. Buying from your local farmer strengthens your community and gives you the opportunity to exert some influence on the quality of your food with your buying decisions. Buying local also means getting more into eating seasonally which is also a good idea.

Plant-Based

Your body is designed in every way to eat plant-based foods. Your teeth, jaws, tongue, shape of you face, length of your digestive tract, saliva pH, stomach pH, blood pH, even your feet, hands, speed and agility are all optimized for gathering, consuming, digesting, and absorbing plants not animals. Your body is solar powered, once removed. All life on this planet comes from the sun. Only plants can transform the sun's energy into carbohydrates through the process of photosynthesis. When we eat plants and drink plant juices it is like we are eating and drinking sunshine! When we attempt to eat animal flesh we are getting our nutrition from an inferior and burdensome secondary source compared to the primary source (plants.) We have a much harder time digesting flesh and it brings along with it toxins, cholesterol, and parasites with which we cannot cope. This leads to metabolic acidosis, weakness, mental fog, sickness, disease and shortened lifespan. In order to eat animals we need all kinds of artificial tools such as traps, guns, knives, etc. No such accoutrements are needed to gather plant foods. It is way easier to sneak up on a head of lettuce than it is a rabbit!

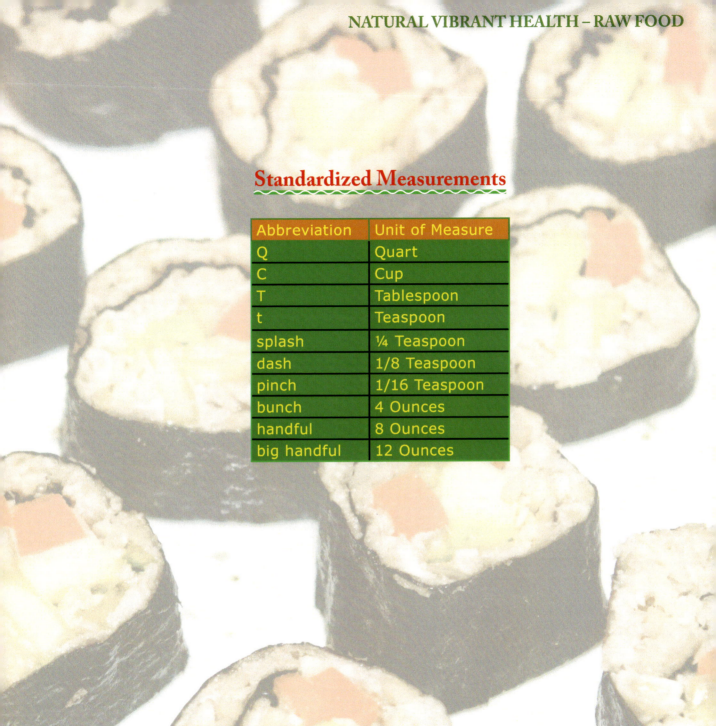

NATURAL VIBRANT HEALTH – RAW FOOD

Standardized Measurements

Abbreviation	Unit of Measure
Q	Quart
C	Cup
T	Tablespoon
t	Teaspoon
splash	¼ Teaspoon
dash	1/8 Teaspoon
pinch	1/16 Teaspoon
bunch	4 Ounces
handful	8 Ounces
big handful	12 Ounces

RECIPES FOR LIVING

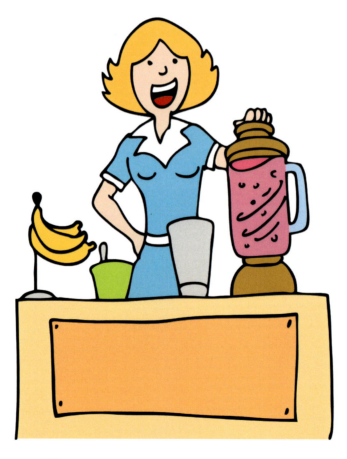

24 - *Raw Food* – NATURAL VIBRANT HEALTH

Smoothies

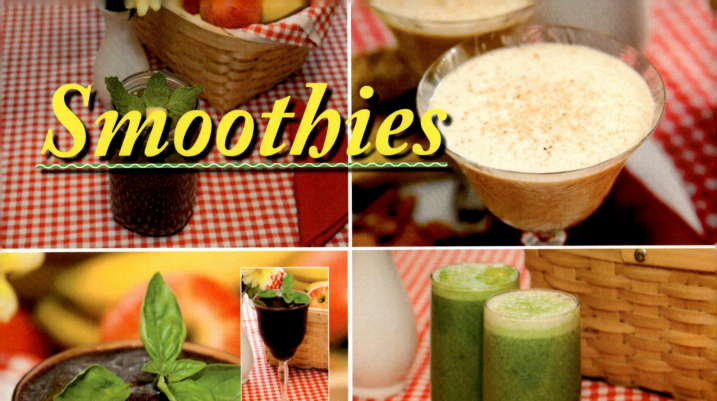

Reasons to drink green smoothies!!!

Green smoothies are tasty for both adults and children.

Green smoothies reduce cravings for sugar and other processed foods that are not good for you.

The fiber in green smoothies helps improve elimination.

Green smoothies can help you lose weight and can give you beautiful skin, bright eyes, and shiny hair.

You will experience overall improved health, increased energy and clearer thinking when consuming green smoothies on a regular basis.

Green smoothies are easy to digest.

Green smoothies are easy to make, and quick to clean up after.

"We always start off our raw food "cooking" classes with a green smoothie! This is because they are the easiest way to get more greens into the diet. Greens are loaded with minerals which are essential for optimal health. Blending the greens with fruit makes them taste better! Plus, blending opens up the cell walls of the greens, making their nutritional constituents easier for your body to assimilate. We recommend a green smoothie every day in addition to a high fiber, high water content diet. You could live on green smoothies."

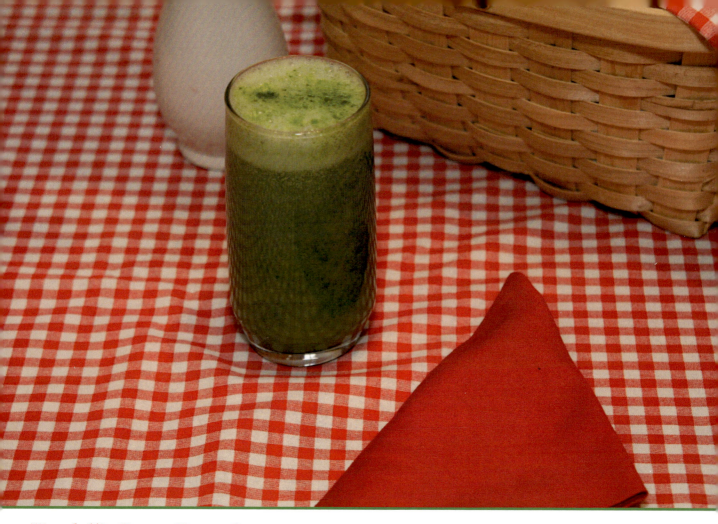

Kendell's Green Smoothie

1 stalk celery	**Sodium**	Stiff Joints
2 C coconut water	**Electrolytes**	Heart
½ cucumber	**Silica**	Myofascial Tissue
1 banana	**Potassium**	Blood Pressure
1 champagne mango	**Vitamin A**	Eyes
1 avocado	**Carotenoid Lutein**	Eyes
1 handful spinach	**Iron**	Anemia
1 t green powder	**Minerals**	Tissue Development
2 T protein powder*	**Amino Acids**	Muscles

* we recommend Sun Warrior Protein Powder.

Combine all ingredients in a blender and blend thoroughly. You can also substitute collard greens, kale or swiss chard for the spinach.

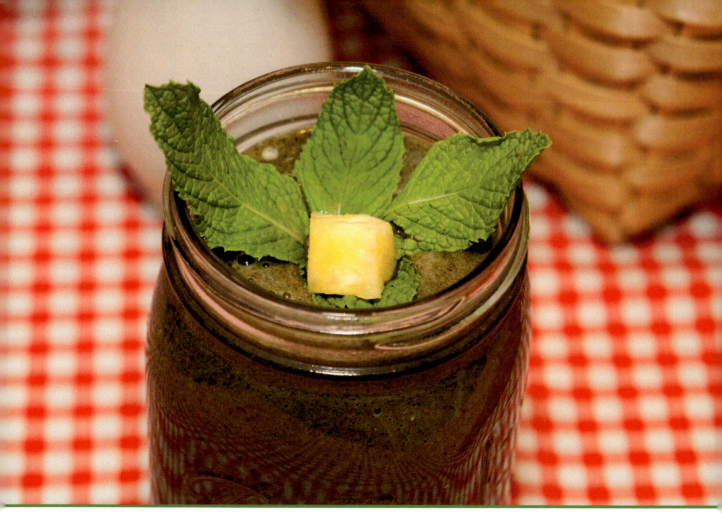

Super-Power Smoothie

2 C coconut water	**Electrolytes**	Heart
1 banana	**Potassium**	Blood Pressure
2 T cacao powder	**Magnesium**	Nerves
1 T coconut oil	**Lauric Acid**	Hair
½ t blue-green algae	**Protein**	Muscles
¼ t cordyceps	**Natural Killer Cells**	Immune System
1 T goji berries	**Antioxidants**	Anti Aging
1 T maca powder	**Testosterone**	Hormones
2 T protein powder*	**Amino Acids**	Muscles

* we recommend Sun Warrior Protein Powder.

Combine all ingredients in a blender and blend thoroughly.

Watch Out!!

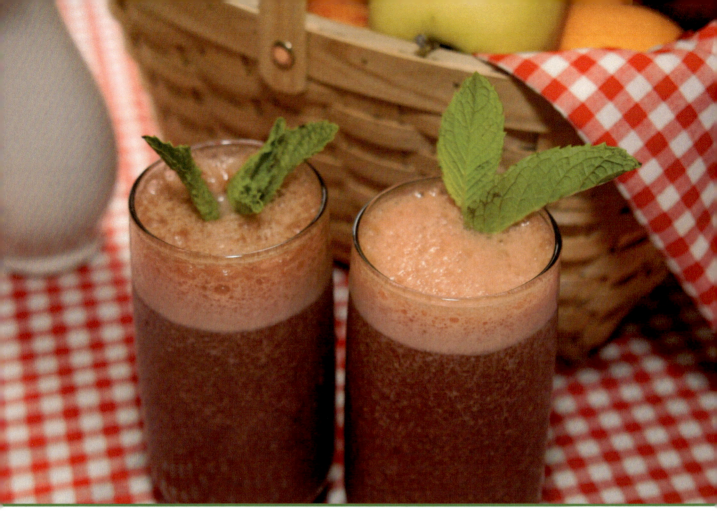

Cherry-Fire Smoothie

½ banana
1 apple
1 C frozen organic cherries
2 C coconut water
1 handful goji berries
½ t cayenne powder

Potassium — Blood Pressure
Antioxidants — Anti Aging
Vitamin C — Immune System
Electrolytes — Heart
Antioxidants — Anti Aging
Capsaicin — Cardiovascular

Combine all ingredients in a blender and blend thoroughly.

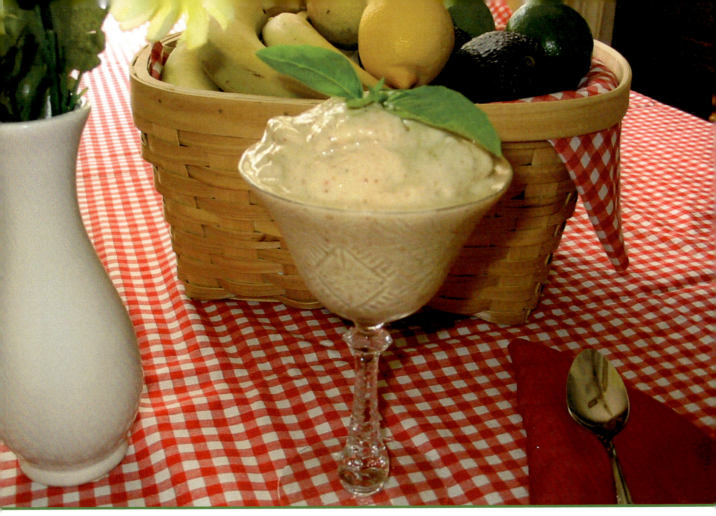

Memory Nut Nog

4 C almond milk (see page 30)	**Calcium**	Bones
3 bananas	**Potassium**	Blood Pressure
1 t cinnamon	**Manganese**	Memory
¼ C dates*	**Antioxidants**	Anti Aging
½ t nutmeg	**Myristicin**	Memory
¼ t turmeric	**Curcumin**	Memory
1 t vanilla extract	**Vanilloid**	Aphrodisiac

* The dates should be soaked for 20 min.

Put all ingredients in a blender and blend well. Makes about 4 servings.

RECIPES FOR LIVING – *Raw Food*

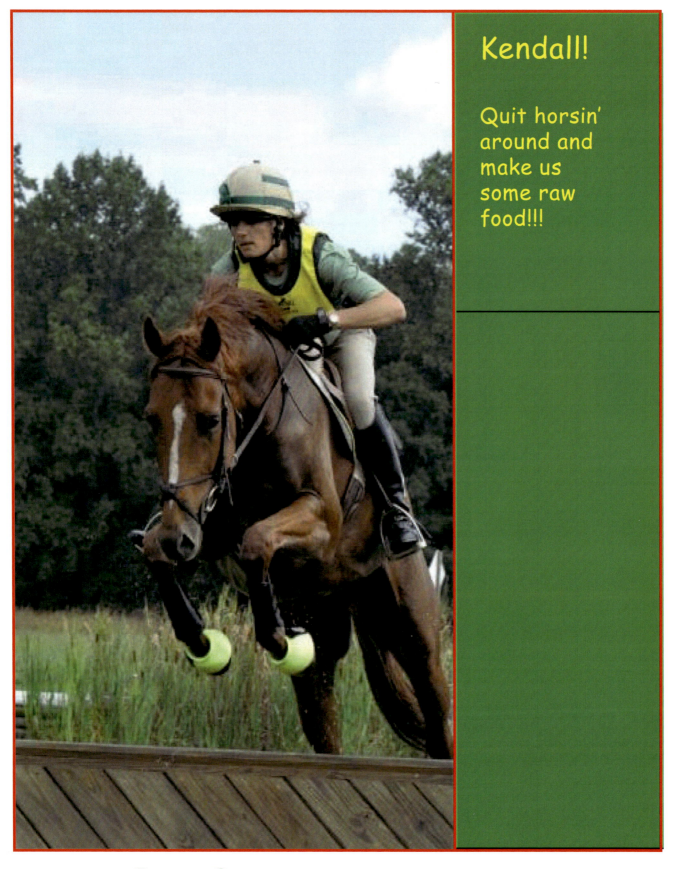

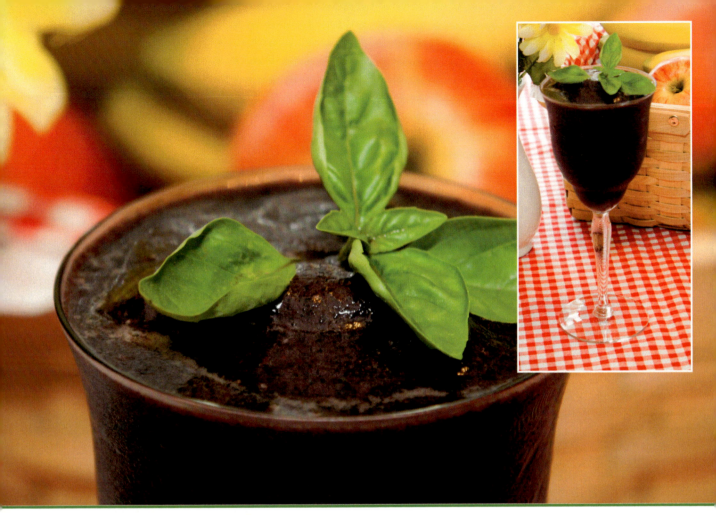

Blueberry Basil Smoothie

12 oz frozen blueberries
2 bananas
1 bunch fresh basil
2 pinches himalayan salt

Antioxidants
Potassium
Vitamin K
Electrolytes

Anti Aging
Blood Pressure
Bones
Nerves

Blend. Add a small amount of water only if necessary. Meant to eat with a spoon.

RECIPES FOR LIVING – *Raw Food*

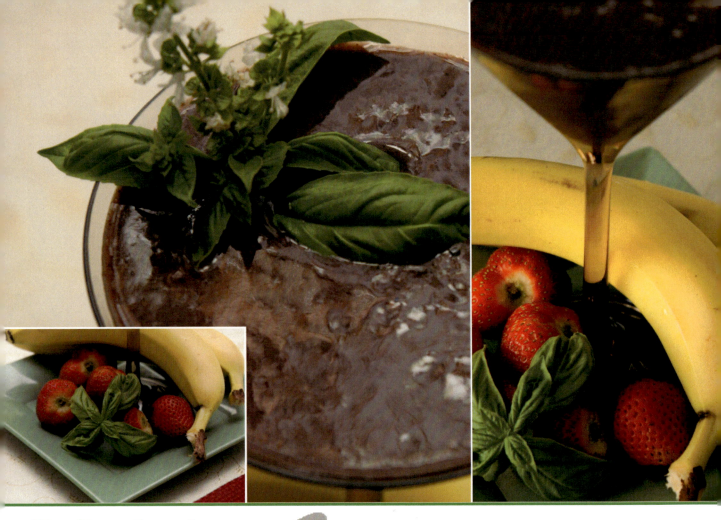

Very Berry Smoothie

2 bananas
1 C strawberries
1 C blueberries
1 big handful of spinach
1 C water

Potassium — Blood Pressure
Folate — Heart
Antioxidants — Anti Aging
Iron — Blood
Oxygen — Cell Respiration

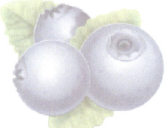

Combine all ingredients in a blender and blend thoroughly.

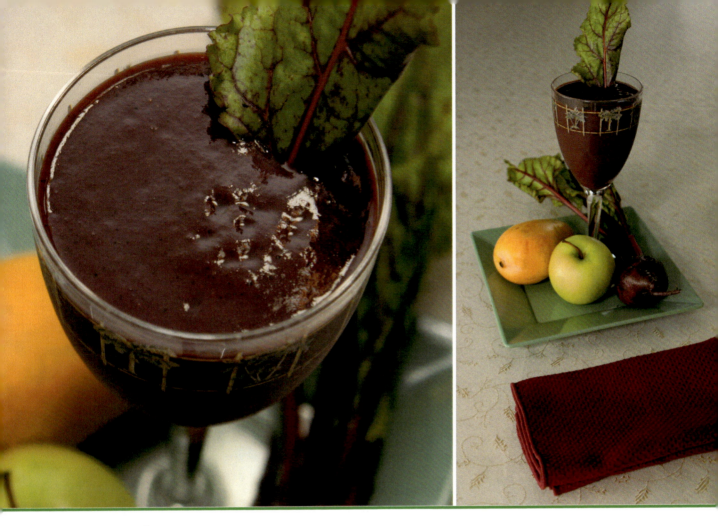

Blue Smoothie

1 bunch beet tops
1 C blueberries
1 champagne mango
1 green apple
1 C water

Manganese   Blood
Antioxidants   Anti Aging
Vitamin A   Eyes
Antioxidants   Anti Aging
Oxygen   Cell Respiration

Combine all ingredients in a blender and blend thoroughly.

RECIPES FOR LIVING – *Raw Food* - 33

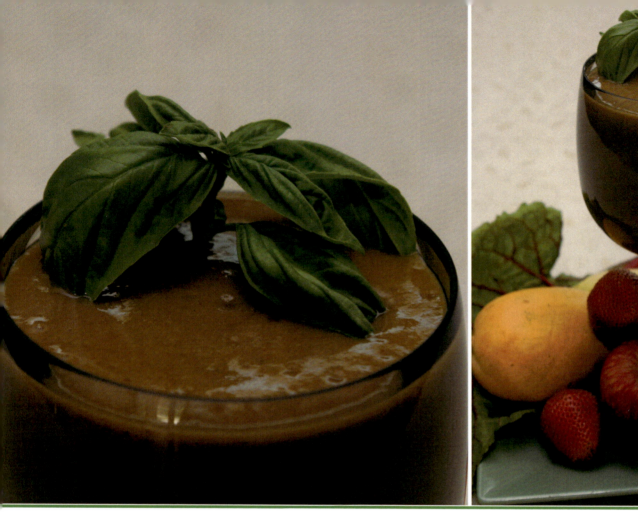

Fruit Chard Smoothie

1 big handful of swiss chard	**Magnesium**	Bones
2 ripe mangos	**Potassium**	Blood Pressure
1 apple	**Antioxidants**	Anti Aging
1 banana	**Potassium**	Stress
1 C strawberries	**Folate**	Heart
6 ice cubes	**Oxygen**	Cell Respiration
1 C water	**Oxygen**	Cell Respiration

Combine all ingredients in a blender and blend thoroughly.

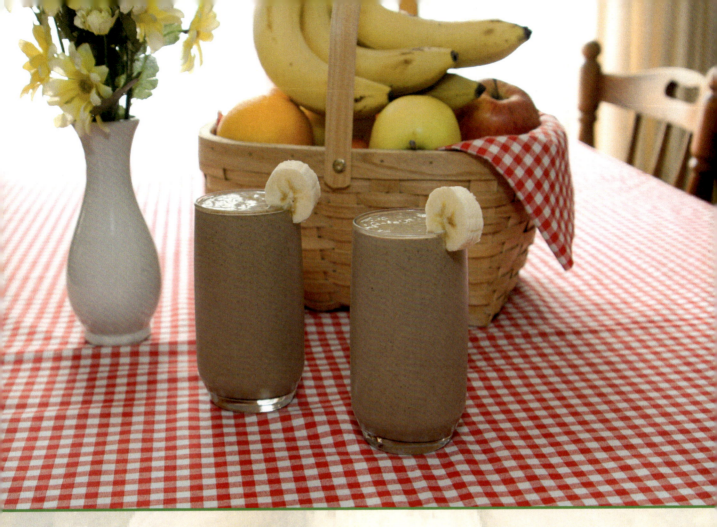

Mocha Chocolate Milkshake

½ C almonds	**Calcium**	Bones
½ C walnuts	**Vitamin E**	Brain
4 medjool dates	**Antioxidants**	Anti Aging
1 frozen banana	**Potassium**	Blood
2 T cacao powder	**Magnesium**	Muscles
2 T Teeccino®	**Prebiotic, Inulin**	Digestive
½ vanilla bean	**Vanilloid**	Aphrodisiac
2 T raw agave	**Inulin**	Cardiovascular
1 pinch himalayan salt	**Electrolytes**	Nerves
3 C ice cubes	**Oxygen**	Cell Respiration
2 C water	**Oxygen**	Cell Respiration

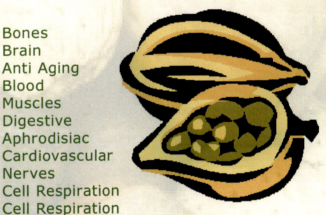

Combine all ingredients in a blender and blend thoroughly.

RECIPES FOR LIVING – *Raw Food*

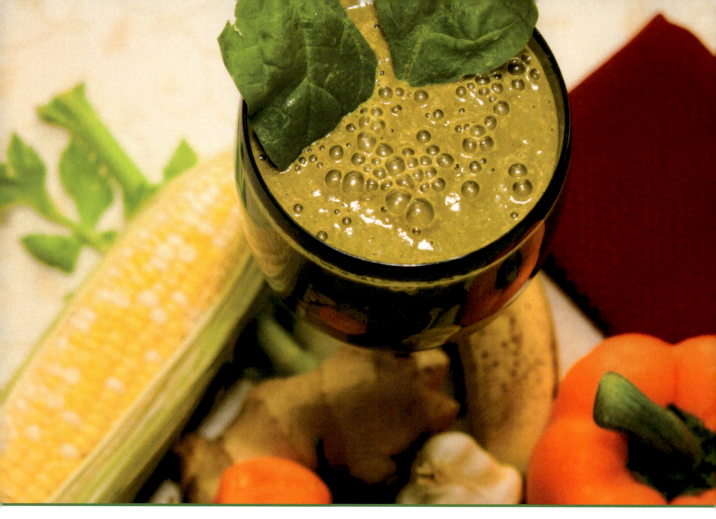

Ultimate Smoothie

2 T goji berries	**Antioxidants**	Anti Aging
1 T cacao powder	**Magnesium**	Nerves
2 T almonds	**Calcium**	Bones
1 T coconut oil	**Lauric Acid**	Immune System
1 T coconut flakes	**Lauric Acid**	Immune System
1 T hemp seeds	**Amino Acids**	Muscles
2 pinches himalayan salt	**Electrolyte**	Nerves
¼ t cayenne powder	**Capsaicin**	Endorphins
1 stalk celery	**Sodium**	Joints
1 clove garlic	**Allicin**	Antibiotic
1 T flax seeds	**Essential Fatty Acids**	Hair
1 carrot	**Vitamin A**	Eyes
¼ red bell pepper	**Vitamin C**	Immune System
½ t cordyceps	**Nucleosides**	Aphrodisiac
1 thimble sized pc of ginger	**Gingerols**	Digestion
3 C spinach	**Iron**	Blood
1 T mesquite powder	**Lysine**	Collagen Formation
1 T maca powder	**Testosterone**	Hormones

NATURAL VIBRANT HEALTH – RAW FOOD

1 t blue-green algae	**Protein**	Muscles
2 bananas	**Potassium**	Stress
½ cucumber	**Silica**	Myofascial Tissue
1 ½ C water	**Oxygen**	Cell Respiration
8 ice cubes	**Oxygen**	Cell Respiration

Combine all ingredients in a blender and blend thoroughly. Get ready to blast off!

Maca Blast

2 bananas	**Potassium**	Blood Pressure
½ C dates	**Antioxidants**	Anti Aging
1 T maca powder	**Testosterone**	Hormones
1 T cacao powder	**Magnesium**	Nerves
2 T coconut oil	**Lauric Acid**	Hair
2 C almond milk	**Calcium**	Bones
1 pinch himalayan salt	**Electrolytes**	Nerves

Combine all ingredients in a blender and blend thoroughly.

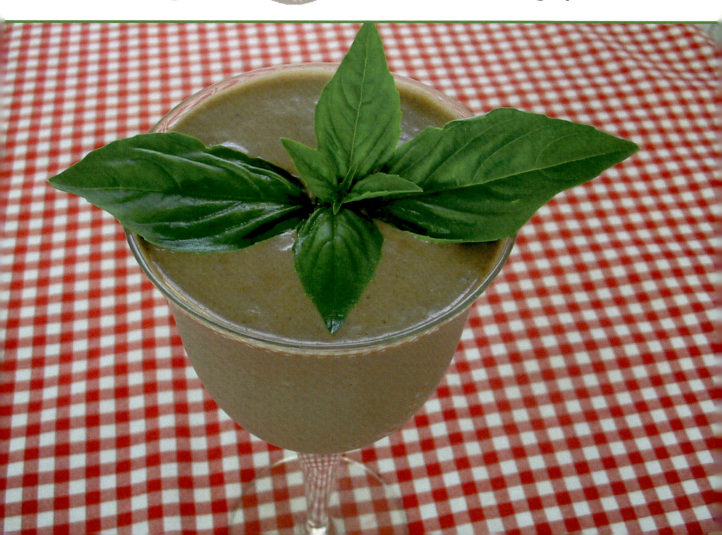

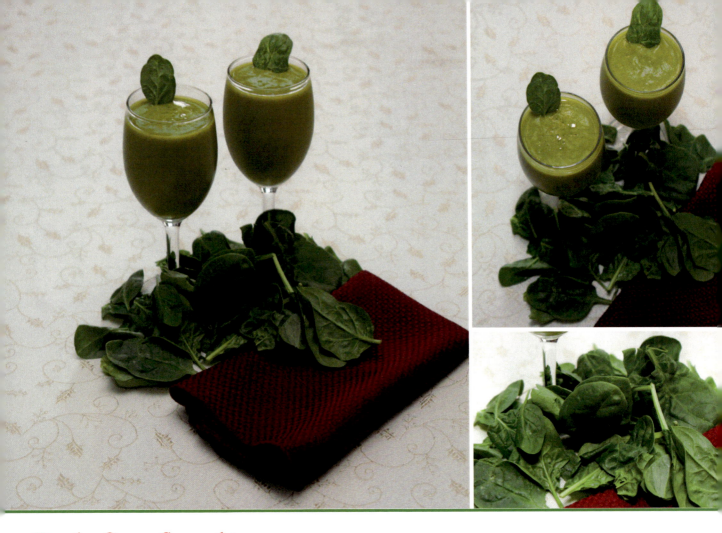

Peachy Green Smoothie

2 handfuls of spinach leaves
6 peaches
1-1/2 C water
6 ice cubes

Iron — Blood
Phosphorous — Skin
Oxygen — Cell Respiration
Oxygen — Cell Respiration

Combine all ingredients in a blender and blend thoroughly.

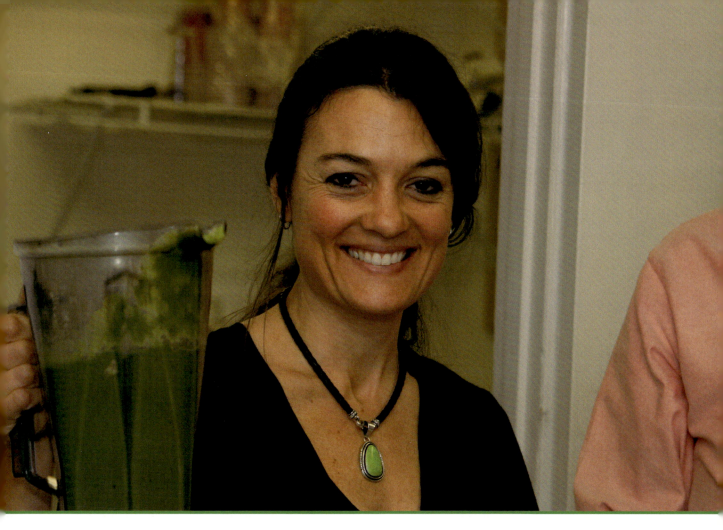

Kale Smoothie

1 big handful of kale
2 bananas
1 C strawberries
½ C pineapple
½ C frozen cherries
1 heaping T cacao powder (optional)
1 C water

Calcium
Potassium
Folate
Bromelain
Vitamin C
Magnesium
Oxygen

Bones
Stress
Heart
Arthritis
Immune System
Muscles
Cell Respiration

Combine all ingredients in a blender and blend thoroughly.

RECIPES FOR LIVING

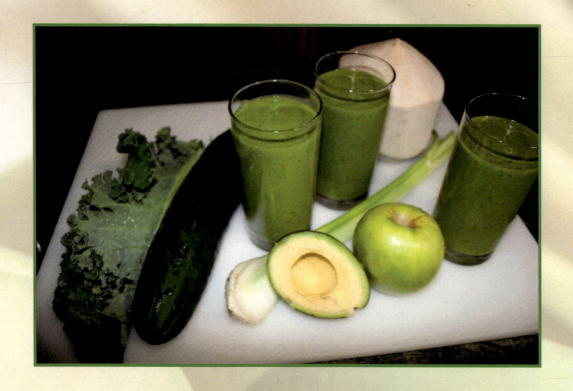

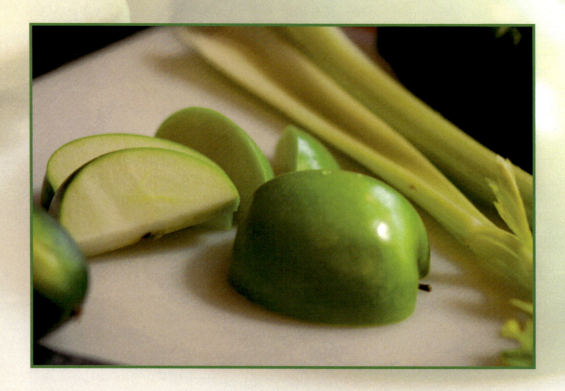

40 - *Raw Food* – NATURAL VIBRANT HEALTH

Drinks & Juices

Fresh made juices are the most potent form of nutrition. When we juice the fruits and vegetables, their goodness is released from the fiber and we are able to drink their highly concentrated nutrients which are then able to enter our bloodstream very quickly. Since juicing removes the indigestible fiber, nutrients are available to the body in much larger quantities than if the piece of fruit or vegetable was eaten whole. For example, because many of the nutrients are trapped in the fiber, when you eat a raw carrot, you are only able to assimilate about 1% of the available beta carotene. When a carrot is juiced, removing the fiber, nearly 100% of the beta carotene can be assimilated. Green juices are the best, like wheatgrass juice. They provide your blood and body with the essential nutrients and purification that they require. Fresh green juices provide us with minerals, vitamins, essential fatty acids, carbohydrates, proteins and much more. The nutritional essence of plants is best derived from their juice. Sunlight infuses all life; plants are the storehouses of nature's captured and distributed sunlight. Try to drink at least one green juice a day for optimal health. The only reason we cannot live entirely on juices is because, eventually our kidneys would get tired (after maybe six months of nothing but juices). The kidneys are not designed to carry 100% of the burden of supplying nutrients to the body over a long period of time. However, a short term juice fast is the best remedy for colds and flu's. This supplies nutrients and removes the burden of digestion of fiber which saves energy that can then be used to heal the body.

Here are more reasons to drink Juice!!!

**Cleansing your body of toxins,
Strengthened immune system,
Increased energy,
Increased strength,
Clearing your mind,
Hydration,
Anti Aging,
Glowing complexion,
Stronger bones,
An excellent vehicle for fasting,
Building and maintenance of the electrolyte, kidney and respiratory systems.**

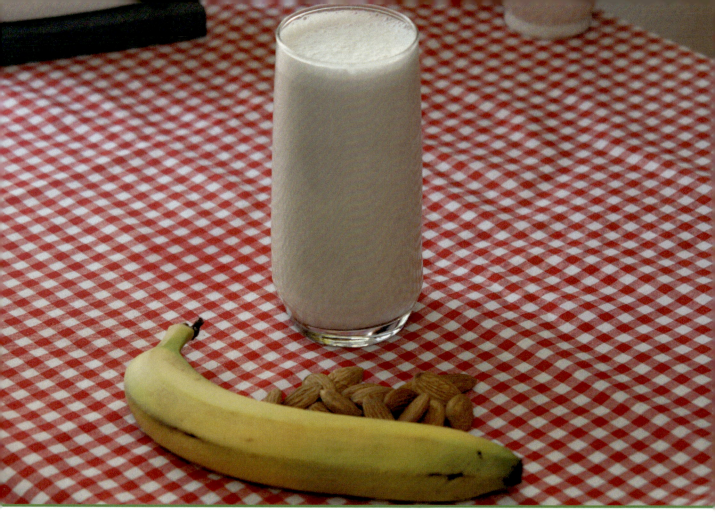

Almond Milk

1 C almonds, soaked and rinsed
1 t vanilla extract
4 C water
1/8 t sea salt

Calcium   Bones
Vanilloid   Aphrodisiac
Oxygen   Cell Respiration

Combine all ingredients in a blender and blend thoroughly. Strain mixture through a nut milk bag into a large bowl. I also like to leave the pulp or use it for other ingredients such as flax crackers. You may adjust the amount of water if you like thicker nut milk or thinner. I like it thicker.

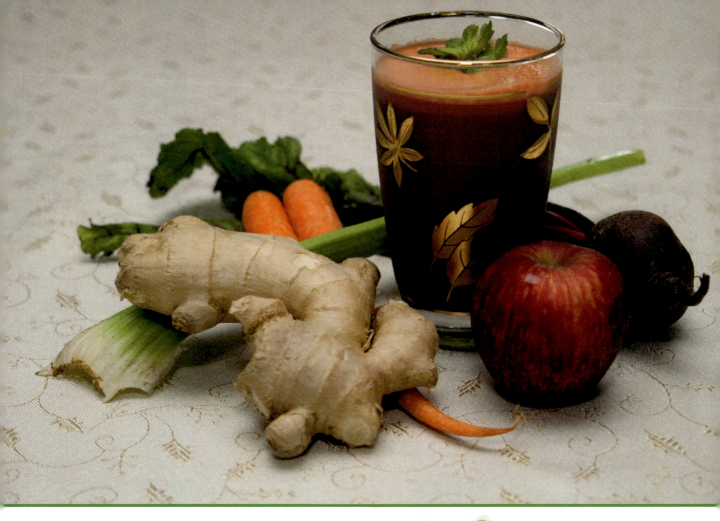

Blood Builder

1 pound carrots
½ beet
2 stalks of celery
1 apple
1 thumbnail sized pc of ginger

Beta Carotene — Eyes
Manganese — Blood
Sodium — Joints
Antioxidants — Anti Aging
Gingerols — Intestines

Place all ingredients in a juicer and juice!

RECIPES FOR LIVING – *Raw Food*

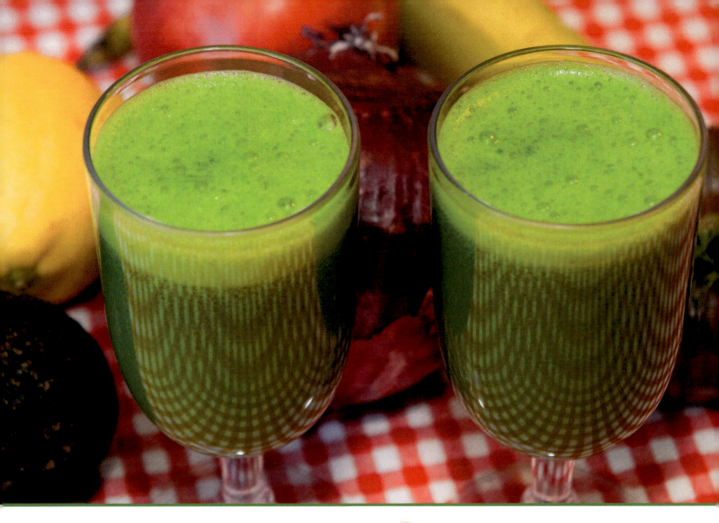

Green Machine

1 cucumber
1 small fistful of parsley
2 stalks of celery
1 piece of kale
1 apple
1 lemon
1 thumbnail-sized pc of ginger

Silica — Myofascial Tissue
Vitamin C — Immune System
Sodium — Joints
Vitamin K — Bones
Antioxidants — Anti Aging
Phytonutrients — Immune System
Gingerols — Digestive

Place all ingredients in a juicer and juice!

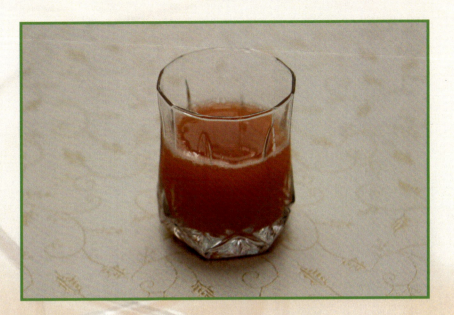

Kombucha

2 Q water
4 raspberry zinger tea bags (or any other preferred flavor)
2/3 C white granulated sugar
½ C Kombucha tea from the last batch you made, or from a friend.
1 SCOBY*

Put water, sugar and teabags into two Mason jars divided equally. Let sit for a few hours in the sun.

Remove tea bags. Add SCOBY and a bit of Kombucha tea, cover with paper towel and the jar lid (rim only.) Let sit at room temperature for a week. Remove SCOBY and ½ cup of the Kombucha tea and set aside for the next batch.

"**SCOBY**" (pronounced "*skoo-bee*". Okay! We may have taken a liberty. But, skoobee sounds so much more fun!)

SCOBY stands for Symbiotic Culture of Bacteria and Yeast. It's what transforms the sweet tea into Kombucha and provides the healthy Probiotics. Here is where you get a Scoby:

>You can get a slice one from a friend who makes Kombucha.
>You can order one through the mail.
>You can grow one from a bottle of store bought Kombucha tea.

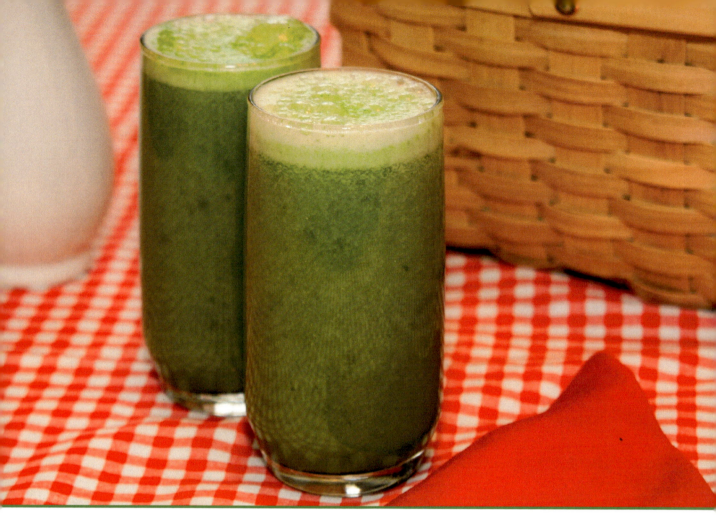

Great Awakenings

½ bunch cilantro	**Vitamin A**	Skin
½ bunch parsley	**Vitamin C**	Immune System
½ bunch arugula	**Vitamin P**	Liver
1 cucumber	**Silica**	Myofascial Tissue
1 apple	**Antioxidants**	Anti Aging
2 celery stalks	**Sodium**	Joints
½ lemon	**Phytonutrients**	Immune System
1 thimble-sized pc of ginger	**Gingerols**	Digestive
½ habanero pepper (WOW!)	**Capsaicin**	Endorphins

Combine all ingredients in a blender and blend thoroughly.

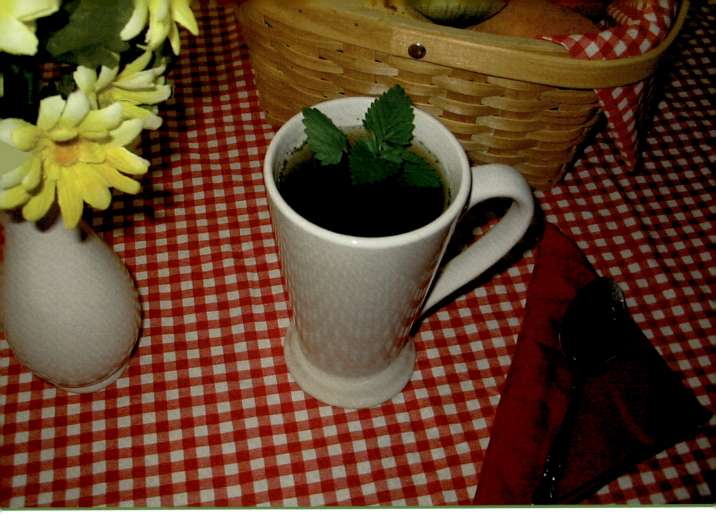

Super Nova Sun Tea

Ginkgo Bilabo	Anti Aging; increases blood flow to the brain; sexual energy
Yohimbe	Increases sexual desire
Anise	Increases sexual desire
Ginseng	Anti Aging; sexual energy; "Fountain of Youth"
Ashwaganda	Sexual capacity and fertility
Astragalus	Metabolism and energy along with stamina
Fenugreek	Phytoestrogens; increased breast size; improved milk production, improves body odor
Rhodiola	Increases serotonin: helping with depression and seasonal affective disorder
Horsetail	Anti Aging; high silica content helps body store calcium; strong tendons, bones
Stinging Nettle	Excellent for allergies. A natural anti-histimine
Goji Berries	Antioxidants; Anti Aging; "Fountain of Youth"
Ho Shu Wu	Hair growth and color, sexual performance

Combine 1 tsp of each in 1 quart water and set in sun for 2 to 4 hours.

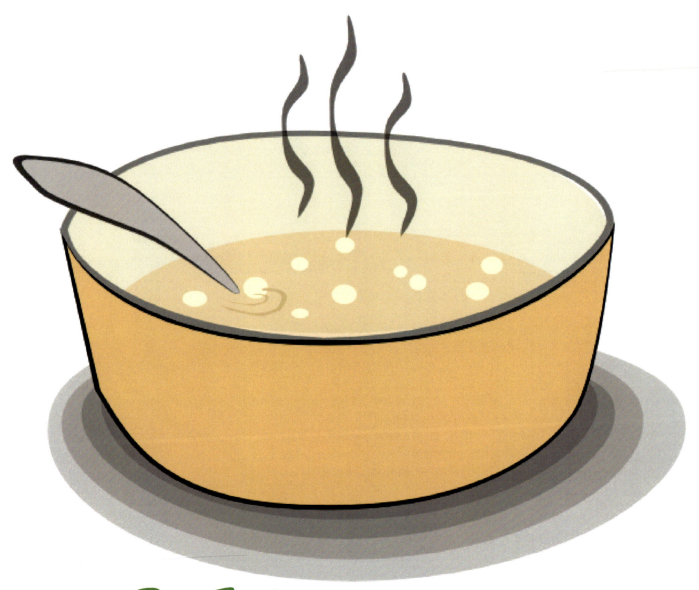

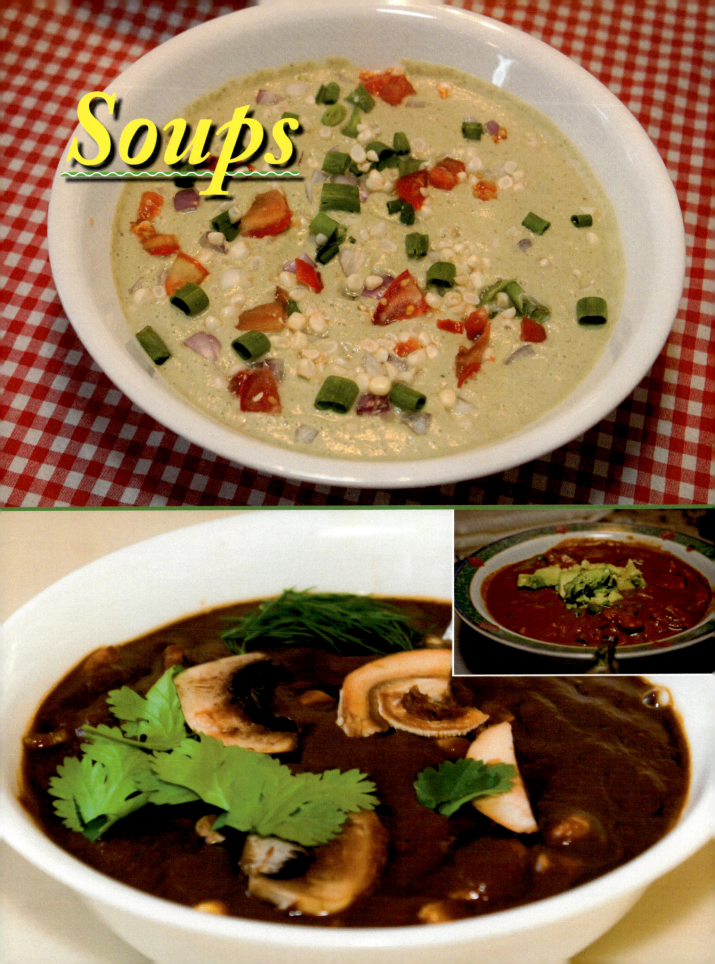

Soups

RECIPES FOR LIVING

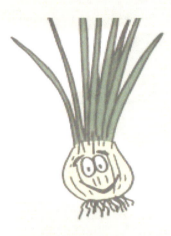

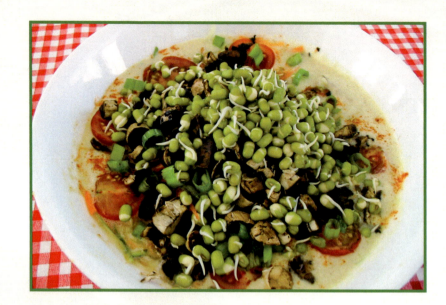

Veggie Miso Soup

Noodles:

½ zucchini
½ cucumber
½ carrot
2 small tomatoes
1 handful mung bean sprouts
1 handful of shitake mushroom

Potassium	Positive Mood
Silica	Myofascial Tissue
Beta Carotene	Eye
Lycopene	Anti Cancer
Protein	Muscle Tissue
Niacin	Memory Power

Soup Base:

3 T miso
½ C extra virgin olive oil
1 thimble sized pc of ginger root
1 clove garlic
2 small shallots
2 C water

Protein	Muscle Tissue
Monounsat Fat	Skin
Gingerols	Digestive
Allicin	Antibiotic
Sulphur	Hair
Oxygen	Cell Respiration

Garnish:

¼ t pepper
parsley
chopped spring onions

Capsaicin	Cardiovascular
Vitamin K	Bone Health
Sulphur	Hair

First, slice the vegetables like noodles using a julienne slicer. Cut the mushrooms into nice bites. Marinate a few hours in olive oil, Nama Shoyu and a little apple cider vinegar. Next, blend the soup base. Take the vegetables out of the marinate sauce and put them in a bowl. Pour the soup base over them and garnish.

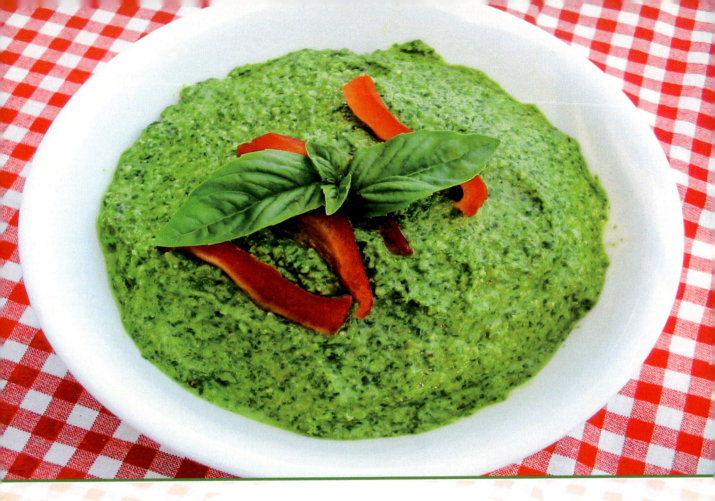

Spinach Curry

½ t himalayan salt
2 T coconut oil
1 t curry powder
2 cloves garlic
1 in. fresh ginger root
2 T lemon juice
½ C macadamia nuts
¼ C chopped onion
4 C chopped spinach

Electrolytes
Antioxidant Lauric Acid
Curcumin
Allicin
Gingerols
Vitamin C
Monounsaturated Fat
Sulphur
Iron

Nerves
Anti Aging
Memory
Antibiotic
Digestive
Immune System
Cardiovascular
Immune System
Anemia

Soak the macadamia nuts or cashews for 4 hours, then rinse. Combine all ingredients in a processor and puree.

RECIPES FOR LIVING – *Raw Food* - 51

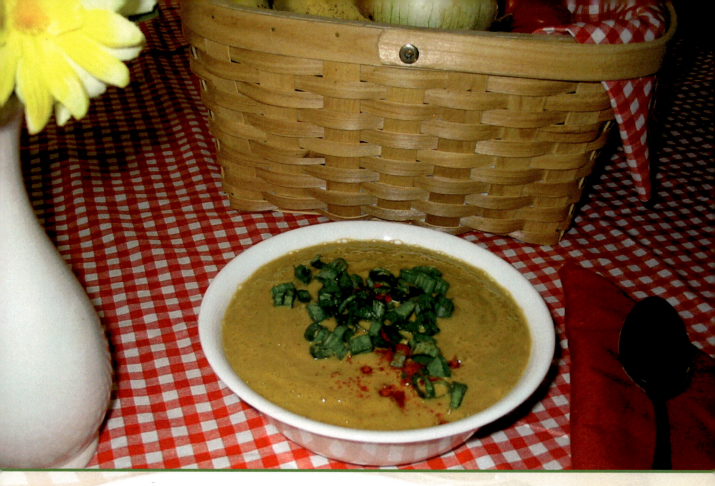

Italian Wedding Soup

1 avocado	**Carotenoid Lutein**	Eyes
4 tomatoes	**Lycopene**	Anti Cancer
1 bunch fresh basil	**Vitamin K**	Blood
1 t miso	**Amino Acids**	Protein
2 scallions	**Sulphur**	Immune System
1 clove garlic	**Allicin**	Antibiotic
¼ C extra virgin olive oil	**Monounsaturated Fat**	Skin
1 T coconut aminos	**Lauric Acid**	Immune System
1 dash cayenne powder	**Capsaicin**	Cardiovascular
¼ C water	**Oxygen**	Cell Respiration

Blend all ingredients.

Garnish:

1 bunch basil leaves	**Vitamin K**	Blood

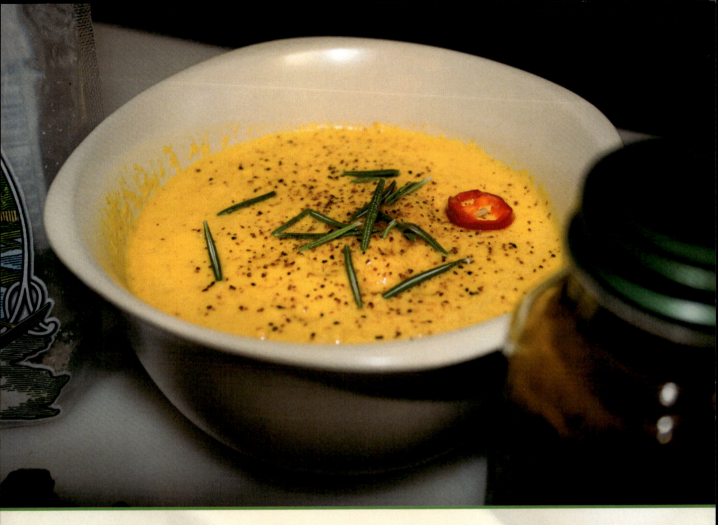

Winter Squash Soup

½ C almond butter
1 butternut squash - peeled, seeded, chopped
½ t himalayan salt
1 T curry powder - I like a little more ☺
1 thimble-sized pc of ginger root
½ t nutmeg
4 C water

Vitamin E — Heart
Carotenes — Antioxidant
Electrolytes — Nerves
Curcumin — Memory
Gingerols — Intestines
Myristicin — Memory
Oxygen — Cell Respiration

Combine all ingredients in a blender and blend thoroughly. Makes about 4 servings. You can substitute acorn squash for the butternut squash.

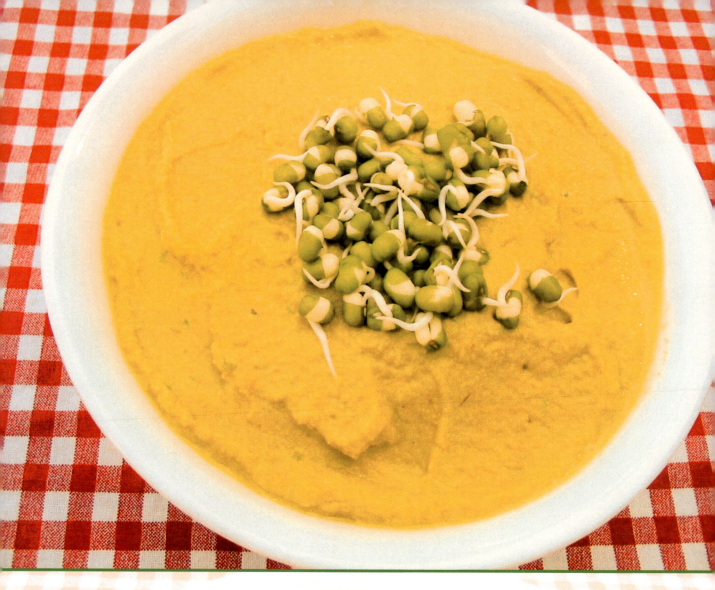

Sweet Potato Soup

1 apple	**Antioxidants**	Anti Aging
1 avocado	**Carotenoid Lutein**	Skin
½ t himalayan salt	**Electrolytes**	Nerves
¼ C coconut meat	**Lauric Acid**	Immune System
¼ C coconut milk	**Lauric Acid**	Immune System
1 C coconut water	**Electrolytes**	Cellular Communication
2 C sweet potato - peeled, chopped	**Carotenoids**	Blood Sugar

Combine all ingredients in a blender and blend thoroughly.

NATURAL VIBRANT HEALTH – RAW FOOD

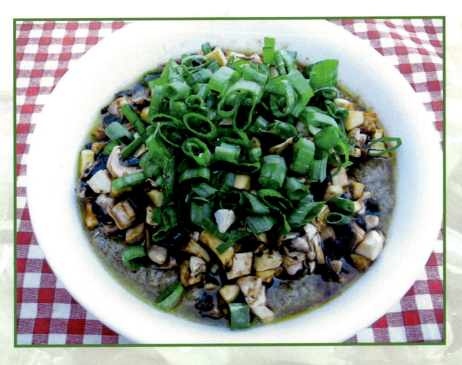
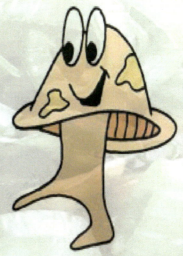

Mushroom Soup

Soup Base:

3 T miso (white or brown)	**Amino Acids**	Protein
1 C extra virgin olive oil	**Monounsaturated Fat**	Skin
1 clove garlic	**Allicin**	Immune System
1 T grated ginger	**Gingerols**	Digestive
½ C portabella mushrooms	**Selenium**	Antioxidant
1 T coconut aminos	**Amino Acids**	Protein

Blend!

Soup Topping:

3 C sliced shitake mushrooms	**Selenium**	Antioxidant
2 T extra virgin olive oil	**Monounsaturated Fat**	Skin
2 T coconut aminos	**Amino Acids**	Protein
1 chopped scallion	**Sulphur**	Immune System

Marinate mushrooms in coconut aminos.

RECIPES FOR LIVING – *Raw Food*

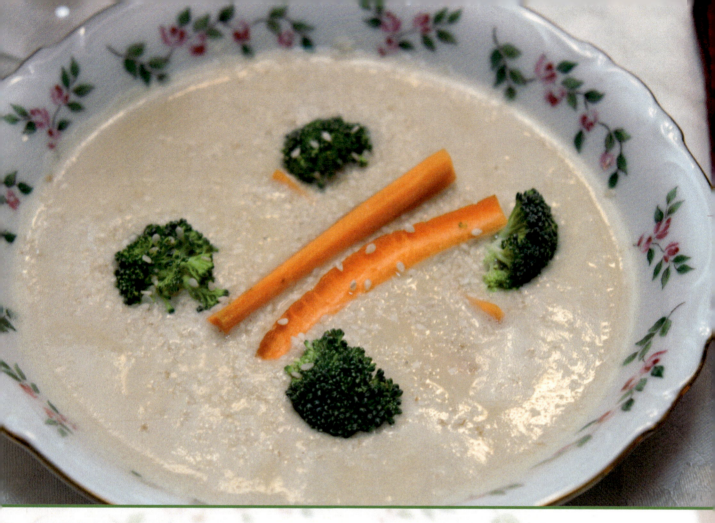

Thai Soup

1 thai coconut (meat & water)	**Lauric Acid**	Immune System
1 T coconut aminos	**Amino Acids**	Protein
1 T miso	**Amino Acids**	Protein
1 T sesame oil	**Essential Fatty Acids**	Cardiovascular
2 T fresh squeezed lemon juice	**Vitamin C**	Immune System
2 T extra virgin olive oil	**Monounsaturated Fat**	Skin
1 t turmeric	**Curcumin**	Memory
½ bunch fresh basil	**Vitamin K**	Blood
2 cloves garlic	**Allicin**	Immune System
1 thimble-sized pc of ginger root	**Gingerols**	Intestines
¼ onion	**Sulphur**	Immune System
1 avocado	**Carotenoid Lutein**	Skin
1 T nutritional yeast	**Lithium**	Blood Pressure
¼ t cayenne powder	**Capsaicin**	Cardiovascular
1 C water	**Oxygen**	Cell Respiration

Combine all ingredients in a blender and blend thoroughly. Makes about 4 servings.

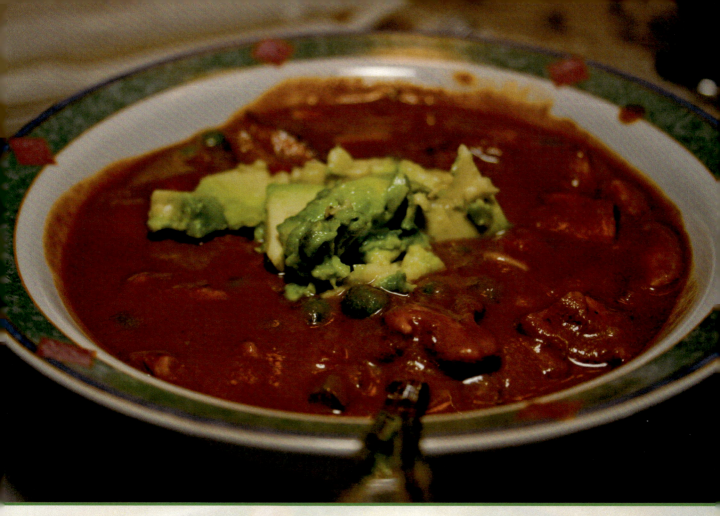

Fiesta Soup

Ingredient	Compound	Benefit
1 thai coconut (meat and water)	**Lauric Acid**	Immune System
½ C soaked sundried tomatoes	**Lycopene**	Anti Cancer
1 T coconut aminos	**Amino Acids**	Protein
1 T miso	**Amino Acids**	Protein
2 T fresh squeezed lemon juice	**Vitamin C**	Immune System
1 T nutrition yeast	**Lithium**	Blood Pressure
2 cloves garlic	**Allicin**	Immune System
¼ onion	**Sulphur**	Immune System
¼ red bell pepper	**Chlorogenic Acid**	Anti Aging
¼ t coriander	**Linoleic Acid**	Anti Arthritic
½ t cumin	**Cuminaldehyde**	Digestion
½ t cilantro	**Cineole Acid**	Chelation
2 T extra virgin olive oil	**Monounsaturated Fat**	Skin
1 C water	**Oxygen**	Cell Respiration
½ t cayenne powder	**Capsaicin**	Cardiovascular

Combine all ingredients in a blender and blend thoroughly. Makes about 4 servings. Garnish with chopped avocado.

RECIPES FOR LIVING – *Raw Food*

RECIPES FOR LIVING

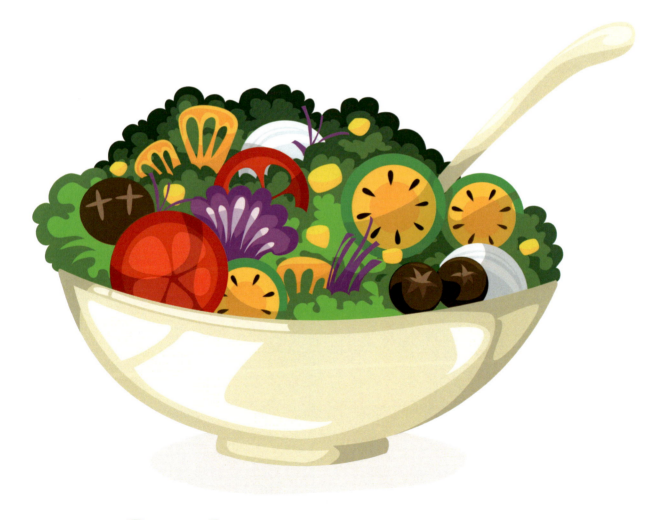

58 - *Raw Food* – NATURAL VIBRANT HEALTH

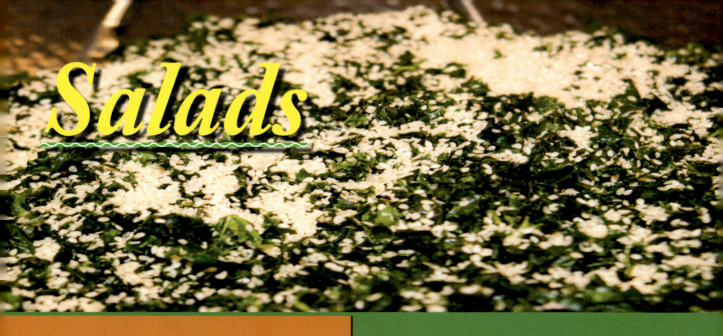

Salads

Where do you get your Calcium!?

Dietary intake of calcium is necessary for healthy bones, teeth, blood and heart. Many people believe that the best dietary source of calcium is from cow's milk. But, is this really true? The fact is, you can get all the calcium you need from plant-based foods as all fruits, nuts, seeds, sprouts, dark leafy greens and vegetables contain calcium. According to the Institute of Medicine (IOM), the daily calcium requirement for men is at least 1000 mg and 1200 mg for women. Here are a few vegan sources of calcium.

Collard Greens	1 cup = 357 mg
Sesame Seeds	¼ cup = 300 mg
Turnip Greens	1 cup = 249 mg
Kale	1 cup = 179 mg
Okra	1 cup = 172 mg
Bok Choy	1 cup = 158 mg
Mustard Greens	1 cup = 152 mg
Tahini	2 Tbs = 128 mg
Broccoli	1 cup = 94 mg
Almond Milk	1 cup = 90 mg
Almonds	¼ cup = 89 mg
Almond Butter	2 Tbs = 86 mg

Humans cannot use the calcium in milk. Since there is no usable calcium, the brain signals the bone matrix to release calcium into the blood. *"The net result is a loss of calcium from the bone matrix."*
-- The Importance of Organic Calcium vs. Inorganic Calcium: The Women's Body's Ability To Recognize and Utilize Calcium
By: Mark J. Occhipinti, M.S., Ph.D., NDc.

For comparison, 1 cup of cow's milk contains 300 mg of calcium. Notice that there is as much or more calcium in ¾ cup of collard greens as there is in one cup of cow's milk. Plus, plant-based sources of calcium have less fat, less calories and zero cholesterol compared to cow's milk.

In most cases the calcium in plant-based foods is in a more absorbable form than the calcium in dairy or other animal products.

This is because of the relatively high phosphorus content in dairy and other animal products which interferes with our body's absorption of calcium.

Also, dairy and other animal products are acid forming as a by-product of its' own digestion, which forces the body to "borrow" calcium from our bones and teeth in order to neutralize this acid reaction. This calcium leaching does not occur when you consume plant-based foods which are alkaline-ash forming. This is why excess consumption of animal protein and dairy is a leading cause of weak bones. Weight bearing exercises are also helpful building strong bones.

Our bodies also need silica and magnesium (in their natural sources) to build calcium in the bones and are also present in our dark leafy greens, especially Nettles and Horsetail. You can find these in health food stores and make teas from them or add to your smoothies. Weight-bearing exercises are also helpful in building strong bones. Keep in mind that animal-based foods are acid forming and plant-based foods are alkaline-forming.

What About Vitamin D?

You do not need to drink cow's milk to get this important nutrient. The best source of vitamin D is sunlight which transforms cholesterol into vitamin D. Spend 20 minutes a day in the sun wearing shorts. Do not wash for 8 hours after sunbathing to allow the vitamin D to absorb. On those days where sunbathing is not convenient you may want to consider supplementing with Kendell's D3 Serum.

Contrary to what you may have been led to believe, you can get more than enough calcium from a plant-based diet. Plants are not only rich in highly absorbable calcium but, they are teaming with many other important nutrients. They are also free of the health concerns, environmental and ethical issues associated with consuming dairy products.

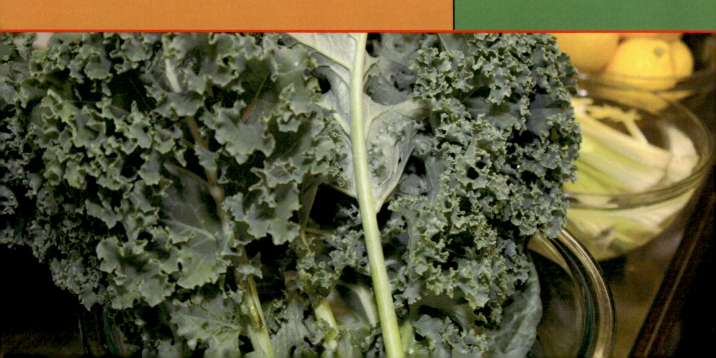

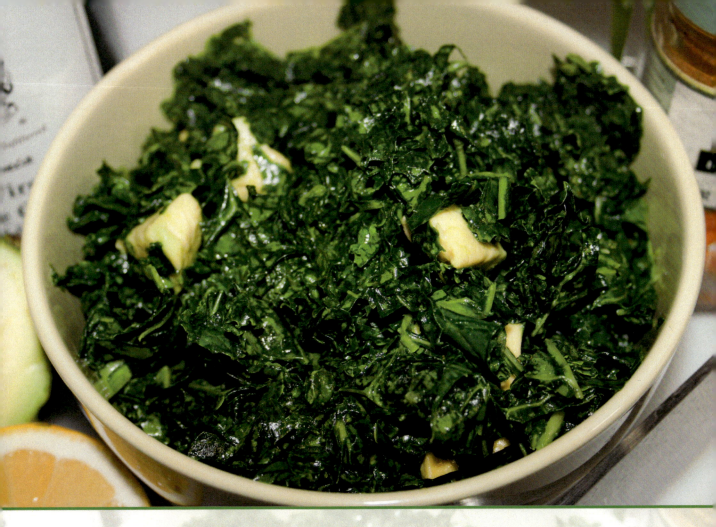

Kale Salad

1 bunch kale de-stemmed	**Calcium**	Bones
1 avocado	**Carotenoid Lutein**	Skin
1 t himalayan salt	**Electrolytes**	Nerves
½ t cayenne powder	**Capsaicin**	Cardiovascular
1 t cumin	**Cuminaldehyde**	Digestion
¼ C lemon juice	**Vitamin C**	Immune System
¼ C extra virgin olive oil	**Monounsaturated Fat**	Skin

Deeply massage all ingredients by hand with love.

RECIPES FOR LIVING

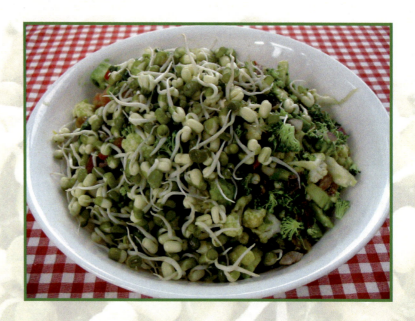

Cauliflower Sprout Salad

Salad:

1 C diced broccoli florets	**Calcium**	Bones
1 C diced cauliflower florets	**Vitamin U**	Digestion
2 diced avocados	**Antioxidant Glutathione**	Anti Aging
¼ C diced red onion	**Sulphur**	Collagen
¼ C chopped basil	**Vitamin K**	Blood
½ C pitted & chopped olives	**Vitamin E**	Cardiovascular
¼ C diced red bell pepper	**Chlorogenic Acid**	Anti Aging

Dressing:

2 ½ T fresh lemon juice	**Vitamin C**	Immune System
3 T extra virgin olive oil	**Monounsaturated Fat**	Skin
1 T coconut aminos	**Amino Acids**	Muscle Tissue

Garnish:

1 C mung bean sprouts	**Zinc**	Prostate

Mix salad ingredients with love in a large bowl and set aside. Combine dressing ingredients in a separate bowl and then pour over salad. Top with garnish.

Entrees & Sides

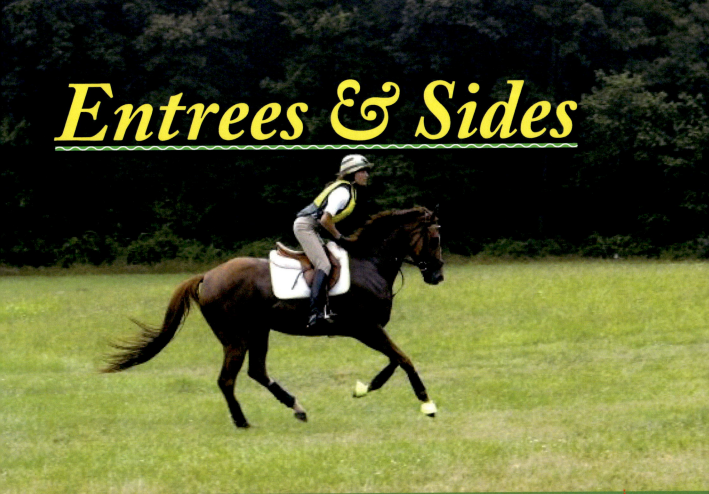

Nice Muscles, Junior!
Where do you get your protein!?

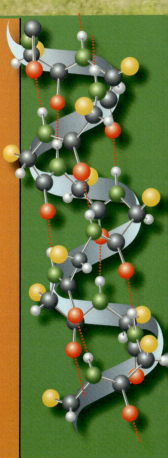

As raw foodists we are frequently asked about dietary sources of protein. This is not surprising since we are all led to believe from an early age that the best way to get protein is by consuming animal products such as beef, chicken, dairy, fish, pork, etc. To some extent, this notion has been carefully nurtured and propagated by certain highly influential special interest groups. There is big money at stake (or, is it steak?) Let's look into the best source of this important nutrient.

Fundamentally, what you really need for muscle and other tissue development is Amino Acids. Amino Acids such as lysine, tryptophan, glutamine, proline and others are the building blocks of the protein molecules. Of the twenty-two Amino Acids, eight are considered "essential" meaning they cannot be synthesized by your body from other compounds and must be taken in as food.

The reality is that all plants contain Amino Acids in abundance. Dark leafy greens, avocados, nuts, seeds and sprouts are a particularly good source of Amino Acids. Plants are actually the best source of protein for humans for the following reasons:

- When you eat plants, the individual Amino Acids are abundantly available and are delivered in their raw, unassembled form. Your body can take exactly the right amount of Amino Acids it needs and build the proper size and shape protein molecules that your body can use to build and replenish muscles and other tissues.

- When you eat animal flesh, protein molecules are delivered in their whole, assembled form. Unfortunately, these animal protein molecules are the wrong size and shape for your body to be able to use directly. Your body must first disassemble these whole protein molecules to break them down into elementary Amino Acids which can then be used to reconstruct new protein molecules in the correct configuration. This takes a lot of extra time and energy. And, this inefficient process also creates a lot of excess waste by-products which becomes a burden on the body.

- Protein and Amino Acids are somewhat heat-sensitive - about half of them are destroyed in the cooking process. Because of this fact, raw foods actually have more available protein/Amino Acids than cooked meat. There is actually more usable and available protein in raw spinach than there is in a T-bone steak!

- Your digestive tract is designed to best digest and assimilate nutrients from plant-based foods. It is long (about 27 feet) like that of other herbivores in nature. This is best for high fiber foods that have a fast transit time. Only plant-based foods contain fiber. Also, your digestive juices are optimized for digesting and assimilating nutrients from plant-based foods.

- Animal-based foods are acid forming and plant-based foods are alkaline-forming.

- There is zero cholesterol in plant based foods.

Where do cattle get their protein?

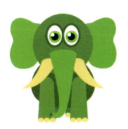

How about gorillas, elephants, giraffes, horses and the rhinoceros? Think about it....these animals are among the largest on the planet and, pound for pound are the strongest, and all they eat are plants! They all get their protein from the Amino Acids contained in plant-based foods, particularly dark, leafy greens.

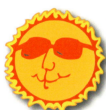

All life energy on this planet comes from the sun. Green plants are the only thing on this planet that can transform the sun's energy directly into the fundamental nutrients that your body can best use. Eating meat takes 100 times more energy out of you than it gives you. When you get your nutrients from animals you are getting them from an inferior secondary source.

There are also many compelling environmental and ethical reasons for getting our nutrients from plants as opposed to animals. Sourcing our food from animals consumes 20 to 50 times the amount of land, water and air compared to nourishing ourselves with plant-based foods. World hunger and much environmental pollution could be eradicated virtually overnight if just a small fraction of carnivorous humans became vegetarians. Other problems with eating animal flesh include the unintentional ingestion of parasites and toxic chemicals in the meat (hormones, steroids, adrenaline, antibiotics, etc.)

Are you anatomically designed to be an herbivore or a carnivore? When it comes to questions like this it is sometimes helpful to forget what you have learned on TV and look to nature for the correct answer. How did the original primal humans eat in the wild? Whenever the bird and the book disagree, always believe the bird. Some things are obvious if you use a little intuition.

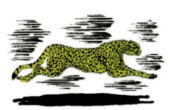

Humans do not have the speed, agility, endurance, claws and fangs to chase and bring down animal prey. If you jumped up onto the back of a cow and tried to take a bite out of her flesh, your teeth would come out of your head and you would only amuse the cow! This is why people are forced to use knives and forks when they attempt to eat animal flesh. Utensils are not needed to eat a peach. It is way easier to sneak up on a head of lettuce then it is to sneak up on a rabbit!

Your best source of protein is actually from plant-based foods, especially dark leafy greens, sprouts, avocados, nuts and seeds. Anatomically and gastronomically you are best suited to acquire your nutrition as an herbivore, not as a carnivore.

RECIPES FOR LIVING

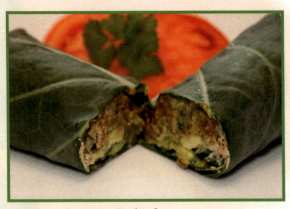

Kendell's Famous Raw Burritos

Cashew Sour Cream

2 C cashews	**Magnesium**	Stress Relief
¼ t himalayan salt	**Electrolytes**	Nerves
1 T nutritional yeast	**Lithium**	Blood Pressure
2 T lemon juice	**Vitamin C**	Immune System

Blend all ingredients in a high speed blender until creamy. You may need to add water as you go.

Guacamole

1 avocado	**Carotenoid Lutein**	Eyes, Skin
¼ t sea salt	**Electrolytes**	Nerves
1 t fresh chopped cilantro	**Cineole, Linoleic Acid**	Anti Arthritic, Rheumatic
½ minced garlic clove	**Allicin**	Antibiotic
1 T lime juice	**Flavonoids**	Skin
1 T chopped onion	**Sulphur**	Immune System

Mix all ingredients together.

Taco Meat

1 t nama shoyu	**Electrolytes**	Nerves
1 T chili powder	**Capsaicin**	Cardiovascular
1 minced garlic clove	**Allicin**	Antibiotic
1 t extra virgin olive oil	**Monounsaturated Fat**	Skin
½ C sundried tomato	**Lycopene**	Anti Cancer
2 C walnuts	**Vitamin E**	Cardiovascular
(soaked overnight)		

Mix all ingredients together in a food processor until it reaches the texture of ground beef. Wrap all the ingredients together in a collard green leaf. You'll be amazed! You can also substitute brazil nuts or pecans in place of the walnuts.

Raw Food – NATURAL VIBRANT HEALTH

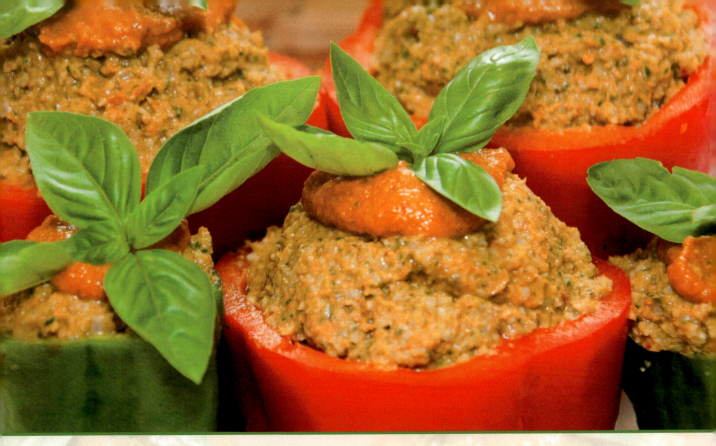

Stuffed Bell Peppers

4 red bell peppers	**Vitamin C**	Immune System
1 C soaked sunflower seeds	**Vitamin E**	Cardiovascular
1 C soaked walnuts	**Vitamin E**	Cardiovascular
3 chopped carrots	**Beta Carotene**	Eyes
1 medium onion	**Sulphur**	Immune System
¼ C medjool dates	**Antioxidants**	Anti Aging
¼ C extra virgin olive oil	**Monounsaturated Fat**	Skin
1 juiced lemon	**Vitamin C**	Immune System
½ bunch fresh basil	**Vitamin K**	Blood
1 t thyme	**Thymol**	Respiratory
1 t himalayan salt	**Electrolytes**	Nerves
1 jalapeno pepper	**Capsaicin**	Cardiovascular
1 t cumin	**Curcumin**	Memory
½ t cayenne powder	**Capsaicin**	Cardiovascular

Chop the tops off of the red bell peppers, hollow out and set aside. Place the sunflower seeds and walnuts in a food processor and grind until fine. Set aside in a separate bowl. Place carrots in the food processor and grind until pureed. Add remaining ingredients to the pureed carrots in the food processor and blend for one to two minutes occasionaly stopping to scrape the sides of the container. Add mixture to the ground nuts and seeds and mix thoroughly. Stuff mixture into red bell peppers. Top with marinara sauce (see spaghetti recipe.)

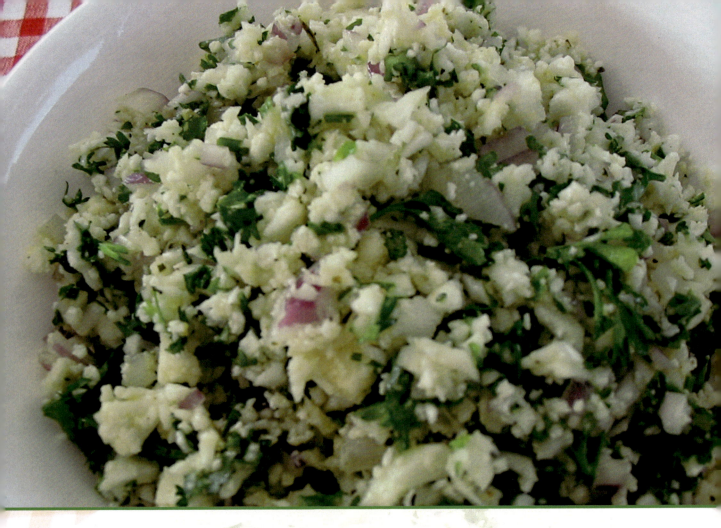

Cauliflower Rice

- 1 C cauliflower
- ½ t sea salt
- ¼ chopped red onion, fine
- ½ C chopped parsley, fine
- ½ t nutritional yeast
- 1 t extra virgin olive oil
- ½ t sage

Vitamin U — Digestion
Electrolytes — Nerves
Sulphur — Immune System
Vitamin C — Immune System
Lithium — Blood Pressure
Monounsaturated Fat — Skin

Place the cauliflower in a food processor and pulse until it reaches the desired texture. Mix remaining ingredients by hands with love in a large mixing bowl.

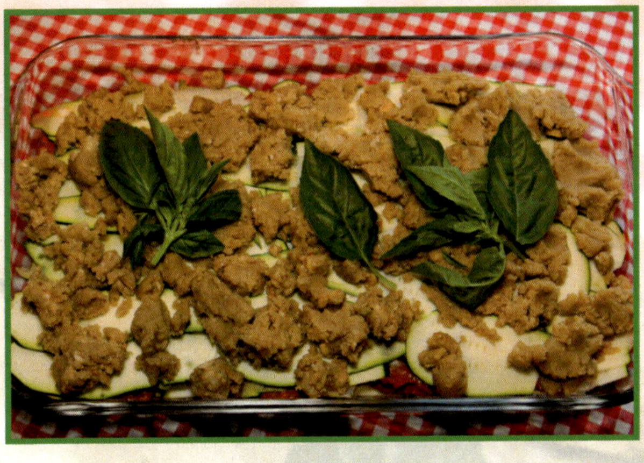

NATURAL VIBRANT HEALTH – RAW FOOD

Lasagna

Noodles

5 zucchinis, thinly sliced using a mandolin
Potassium good for Muscle Tissue

Pesto

2 C raw walnuts
3 oz basil
3 T extra virgin olive oil
1 pinch himalayan salt

Vitamin E — Cardiovascular
Vitamin K — Blood
Monounsaturated Fat — Skin
Electrolytes — Nerves

Blend (use tamper)

Marinara

2 C sundried tomatoes
1 tomato
½ red bell pepper
¼ onion
1 clove garlic
¼ C extra virgin olive oil
1 t crushed red pepper
3 oz oregano
a few leaves of basil
1 pinch himalayan salt

Lycopene — Anti Cancer
Lycopene — Anti Cancer
Vitamin C — Immune System
Sulphur — Immune System
Allicin — Immune System
Monounsaturated Fat — Skin
Capsaicin — Cardiovascular
Antioxidant Carvacrol — Anti Aging
Vitamin K — Blood
Electrolytes — Nerves

Blend (use tamper)

Ricotta

2 C raw cashew, pine or macadamia nuts (soaked 4 hours, then drained)
3 T nutritional yeast
1 lemon juice
1 pinch himalayan salt
¼ C water

Lithium — Blood Pressure
Vitamin C — Immune System
Electrolytes — Nerves
Oxygen — Cell Respiration

Blend/chop in food processor. Alternately layer noodles, pesto, marinara and ricotta.

RECIPES FOR LIVING – *Raw Food* - 69

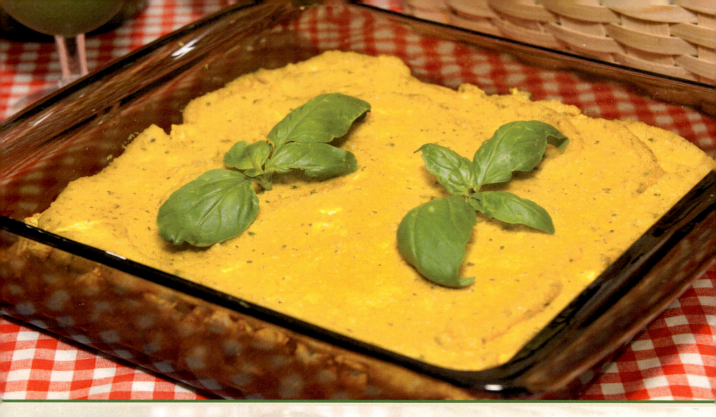

Cheezy Cauliflower Casserole

1 cauliflower head, chopped	**Vitamin U**	Digestion
1 T lemon juice	**Vitamin C**	Immune System
1 T extra virgin olive oil	**Monounsaturated Fat**	Skin
½ t himalayan salt	**Electrolytes**	Nerves
½ t turmeric	**Curcumin**	Memory

Massage all ingredients by hand with love to mix through, and pour cauliflower in casserole dish.

"Cheeze" Sauce Topping

1 C raw soaked cashews	**Copper**	Libido
2 T chopped rosemary	**Choleric**	Antidepressant
2 T extra virgin olive oil	**Monounsaturated Fat**	Skin
2 T lemon juice	**Vitamin C**	Immune System
¼ C water	**Oxygen**	Respiration
3 T nutritional yeast	**Lithium**	Blood Pressure
½ t himalayan salt	**Electrolytes**	Nerves
¼ t cayenne powder	**Capsaicin**	Cardiovascular
½ t turmeric	**Curcumin**	Memory

Blend and pour on top of cauliflower, and then spread evenly.

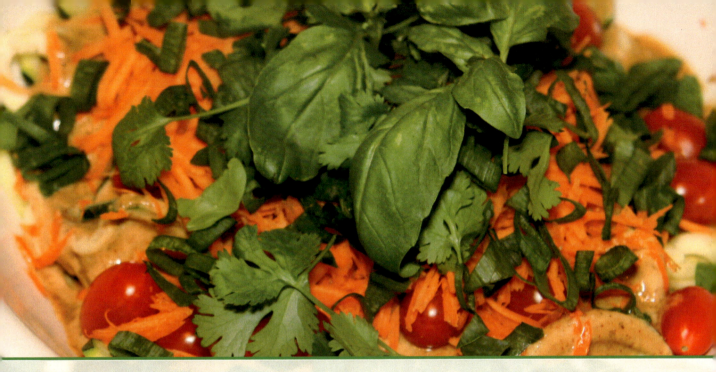

Pad Thai

Sauce

3/4 C raw almond butter	**Vitamin E**	Heart
1/2 C fresh orange juice	**Vitamin C**	Immune System
1 T minced fresh ginger	**Gingerols**	Digestive
1 T coconut aminos	**Amino Acids**	Protein
1 T miso (optional)	**Amino Acids**	Protein
1 t minced garlic	**Allicin**	Antibiotic
2 T raw honey	**Antibacterial**	Immune Strength
1/8 t cayenne powder	**Capsaicin**	Cardiovascular

Blend all ingredients in a food processor or blender until smooth.

Noodles

1 peeled zucchini	**Potassium**	Muscle Tissue

Using a spirooli to create zucchini noodles and then pour the sauce over them to marinate (let them sit for about 10 minutes) and then top them with a mixture of the following:

Toppings

shredded carrots	**Beta Carotene**	Eyes
grape tomatoes	**Lycopene**	Anti Cancer
scallions	**Sulphur**	Immune System
cilantro	**Cineole, Linoleic Acid**	Anti Arthritic, Rheumatic
basil	**Vitamin K**	Blood

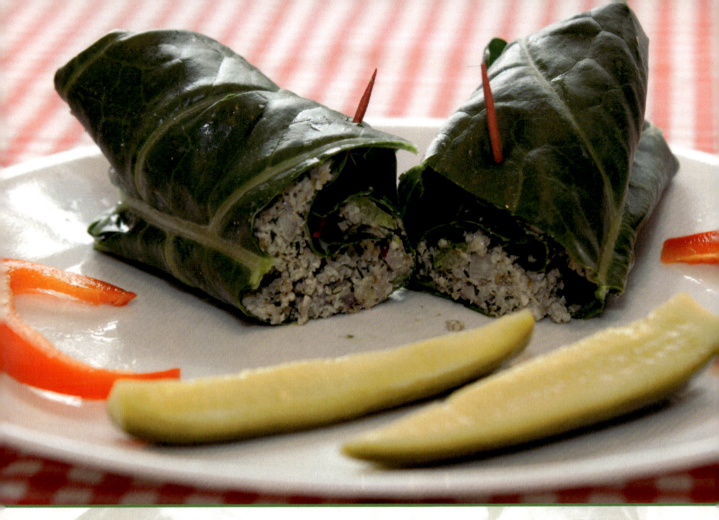

Tuna Wraps

1 C soaked macadamia nuts	**Monounsaturated Fat**	Cardiovascular
1 C soaked sunflower seeds	**Vitamin E**	Cardiovascular
2 T lemon juice	**Vitamin C**	Immune System
1 t mustard powder	**Selenium**	Cardiovascular
1 t himalayan salt	**Electrolytes**	Nerves
½ C dill	**Monoterpenes**	Stress Reduction
¼ C coconut water	**Amino Acids**	Protein
1 clove garlic	**Allicin**	Antibiotic

Process in a food processor. Place in large bowl and mix in:

1 stalk celery, chopped fine	**Sodium**	Stiff Joints
½ red bell pepper, chopped fine	**Vitamin C**	Immune System
½ red onion, chopped fine	**Sulphur**	Immune System
1 chopped raw pickle	**Silica**	Myofascial Tissue

Wrap in large collard leaves.

NATURAL VIBRANT HEALTH – RAW FOOD

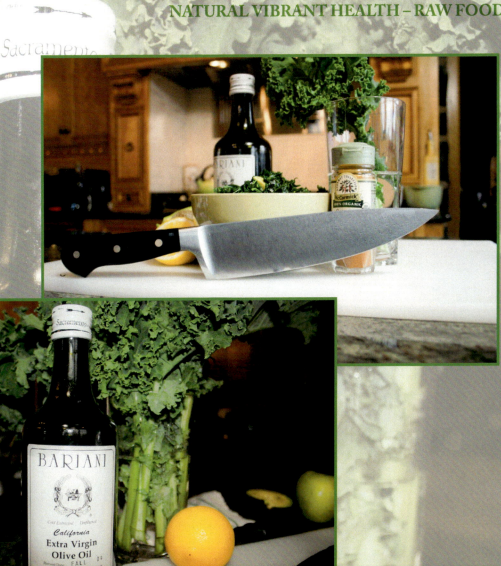

RECIPES FOR LIVING – *Raw Food* - 73

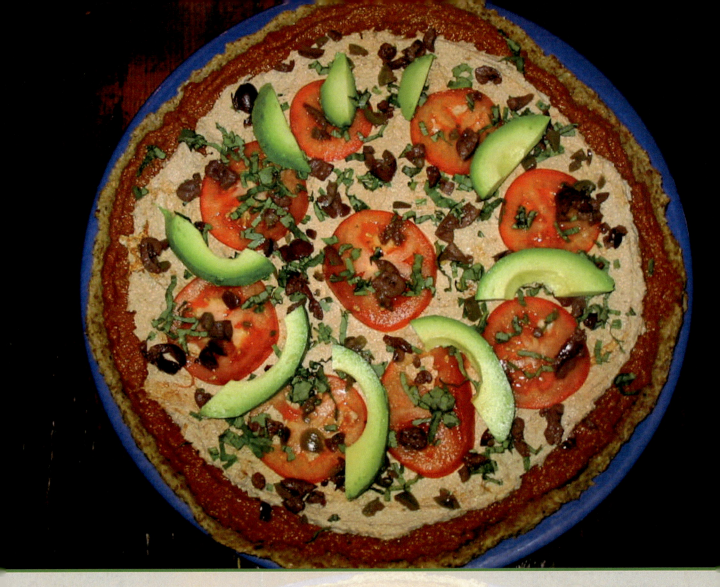

Pizza

Bread

1 C golden flax seeds
½ C coconut aminos
1 C purified water
2 C soaked raw almonds

Omega-3 Fatty Acids — Arthritis
Amino Acids — Protein
Oxygen — Cell Respiration
Calcium — Bones

Process in a food processor. Spread on Teflex sheets on dehydrator trays and dehydrate at 105 degrees F for about 8 hours flipping once and removing Teflex sheets half way through.

NATURAL VIBRANT HEALTH – RAW FOOD

Tomato Sauce

Ingredients	Nutrients	Benefits
2 C sundried tomatoes	Lycopene	Anti Cancer
1 tomato	Lycopene	Anti Cancer
1 red bell pepper	Vitamin C	Immune System
¼ onion	Sulphur	Immune System
2 cloves garlic	Antioxidants	Antibiotic
1 T extra virgin olive oil	Monosaturated Fat	Skin
1 t crushed red pepper	Capsaicin	Cardiovascular
3 oz pkg oregano	Antioxidant Carvacrol	Anti Aging
3 T chopped thyme	Thymol	Respiratory
1 bunch of basil leaves	Vitamin K	Blood
1 pinch himalayan salt	Electrolytes	Nerves

Blend and spread on top of bread.

Cheese

Ingredients	Nutrients	Benefits
2 C raw walnuts, soaked 1 hour	Vitamin E	Cardiovascular
2 T nutritional yeast	Lithium	Blood Pressure
1 T extra virgin olive oil	Monounsaturated Fat	Skin
2 T lemon juice	Vitamin C	Immune System
1 small minced garlic clove	Antioxidant Allicin	Anti Aging
1 T coconut aminos	Amino Acids	Protein
½ C purified water	Oxygen	Cell Respiration

Blend and spread on top. Garnish with sliced avocado, chopped olives, tomatoes and basil.

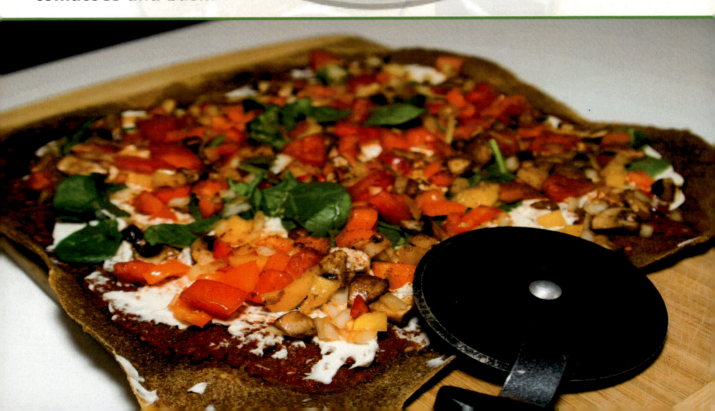

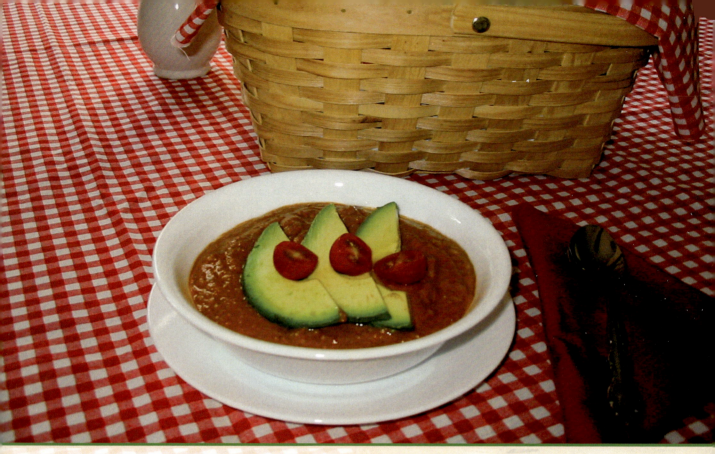

Chili

2 C soaked raw walnuts	**Vitamin E**	Cardiovascular
1 T coconut aminos	**Amino Acids**	Protein
2 cloves garlic	**Antioxidants**	Antibiotic
1 bunch spring onions	**Sulphur**	Immune System
¼ C extra virgin olive oil	**Monounsaturated Fat**	Skin
2 medium sized tomatoes	**Lycopene**	Anti Cancer
1 pkg sundried tomatoes, soaked	**Lycopene**	Anti Cancer
1 red bell pepper	**Vitamin C**	Immune System
2 T thyme	**Thymol**	Respiratory
1 t himalayan salt	**Electrolytes**	Nerves
1 T cumin	**Antioxidants**	Anti Aging
1 T chili powder	**Capsaicin**	Cardiovascular

Place walnuts in a food processor and chop until ground. Place ground walnuts in a mixing bowl. Place remaining ingredients in a blender and blend until smooth. Pour this mixture into the mixing bowl over the ground walnuts and mix well.

Garnish

1 sliced avocado	Carotenoid Lutein	Eyes, Skin
1 handful grape tomatoes	Lycopene	Anti Cancer

Raw Food – NATURAL VIBRANT HEALTH

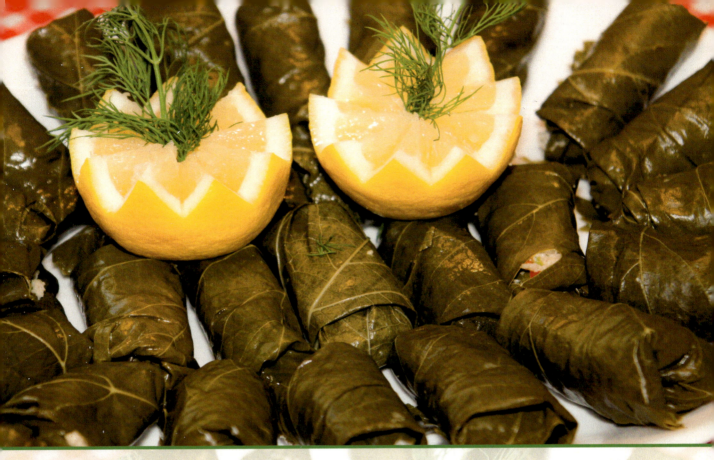

Dolmas

2 C raw sunflower seeds
    (soaked and sprouted)

2 stalks chopped celery
¼ C sundried tomatoes
    (soaked one hour)

4 dates, soaked 30 minutes
1 C basil
1 C dill
2 T dulse
2 T extra virgin olive oil
2 T coconut aminos
1 juiced lemon
24 grape leaves

Vitamin E	Cardiovascular
Sodium	Stiff Joints
Lycopene	Anti Cancer
Antioxidants	Anti Aging
Vitamin K	Blood
Monoterpenes	Stress Reduction
Iodine	Thyroid
Monounsaturated Fat	Skin
Amino Acids	Protein
Vitamin C	Immune System
Niacin	Sleep

Add all ingredients except grape leaves into a food processor and pulse until chunky. Overlap two grape leaves at a time and make a wrap by rolling two heaping tablespoons of filling into the grape leaves tucking in the ends as you go. Dehydrate for four hours.

RECIPES FOR LIVING – *Raw Food*

RECIPES FOR LIVING

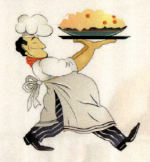
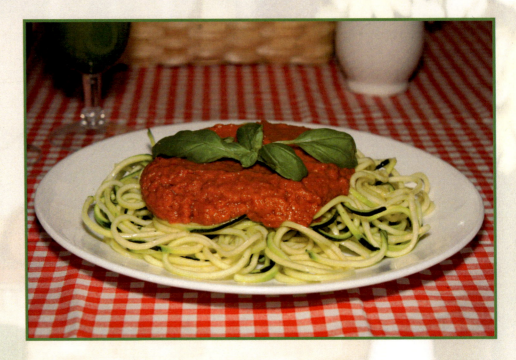

Spaghetti

Pasta

2 zucchinis	**Potassium**	Muscle Tissue
2 T extra virgin olive oil	**Monounsaturated Fat**	Skin
1 pinch himalayan salt	**Electrolytes**	Nerves

Use a spirooli to create zucchini noodles. Place noodles in a large mixing bowl and marinate with salt and olive oil for 15 minutes stirring occasionally.

Marinara

2 C sundried tomatoes	**Lycopene**	Anti Cancer
1 tomato	**Lycopene**	Anti Cancer
1 red bell pepper	**Vitamin C**	Immune System
¼ onion	**Sulphur**	Immune System
2 cloves garlic	**Antioxidants**	Antibiotic
1 T extra virgin olive oil	**Monounsaturated Fat**	Skin
¼ t crushed red pepper	**Capsaicin**	Anti Aging
3 oz pkg oregano	**Antioxidant Carvacrol**	Anti Aging
1 large bunch basil leaves	**Vitamin K**	Blood
1 pinch himalayan salt	**Electrolytes**	Nerves

Top zucchini noodles with marinara and garnish with basil leaves.

Raw Food – NATURAL VIBRANT HEALTH

NATURAL VIBRANT HEALTH – RAW FOOD

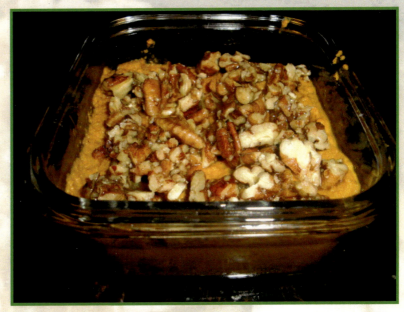

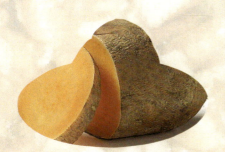

Sweet Potato Casserole

5 raw chopped sweet potatoes	**Carotenoids**	Blood Sugar
1 ½ t cinnamon	**Manganese**	Memory
1 thimble-sized pc ginger	**Gingerols**	Digestion
8 oz soaked dates	**Antioxidants**	Anti Aging
2 C date soak water	**Antioxidants**	Anti Aging
3 oz pecans	**Vitamin E**	Brain
½ t himalayan salt	**Electrolytes**	Nerves

Blend in high speed blender. Pour into casserole dish.

Topping

3 oz pecans	**Vitamin E**	Brain
(smashed with a wooden mallet)		
4 T honey (raw, please)	**Antibacterial**	Immune Strength
½ t himalayan salt	**Electrolytes**	Nerves

Toss and garnish on top of casserole.

RECIPES FOR LIVING

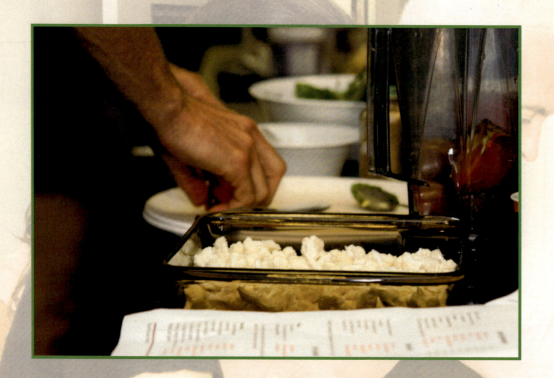

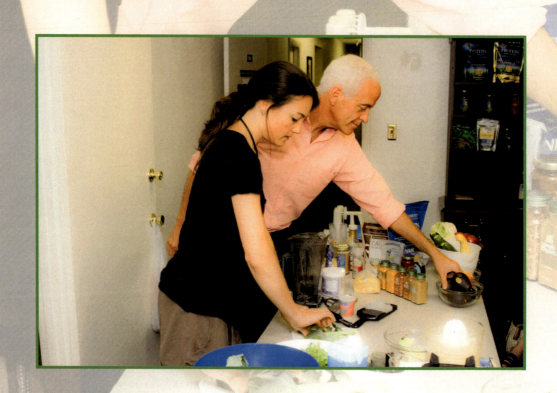

80 - *Raw Food* – NATURAL VIBRANT HEALTH

Burgers

Paté

1 C soaked sunflower seeds
1 C soaked walnuts
3 chopped carrots
1 medium onion
¼ C medjool dates
¼ C extra virgin olive oil
1 juiced lemon
½ bunch basil
1 t thyme
1 t himalayan salt
1 jalapeno pepper
1 t cumin
½ t cayenne powder

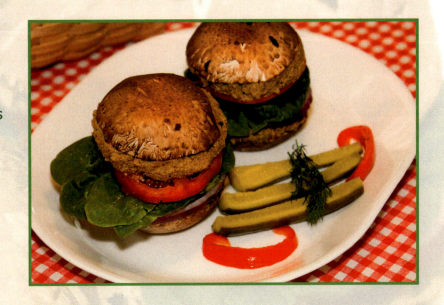

Place the sunflower seeds and walnuts in a food processor and grind until fine. Set aside in a separate bowl. Place carrots in the food processor and grind until pureed. Add remaining ingredients to the pureed carrots in the food processor and blend for one to two minutes occasionaly stopping to scrape the sides of the container. Add mixture to the ground nuts and seeds and mix thoroughly.

Buns

8 large portabella mushrooms

Carefully cut out the mushroom stalks. Place ½ cup of paté in one of the mushroom caps and flatten with a spatula. Garnish with sliced onion, tomato and spinach leaves. Place another ½ cup of paté on top and flatten with a spatula. Garnish with raw ketchup and top off with another mushroom cap.

Ketchup

1 C ripe tomatoes, chopped
1 8 oz jar sundried tomatoes in olive oil
1 sm clove garlic, finely minced
1/4 C raw honey
1 T Bragg's Liquid Aminos®, nama shoyu, or soy sauce
1 T apple cider vinegar

In a blender, puree all ingredients (including all of the oil in the jar of sundried tomatoes).

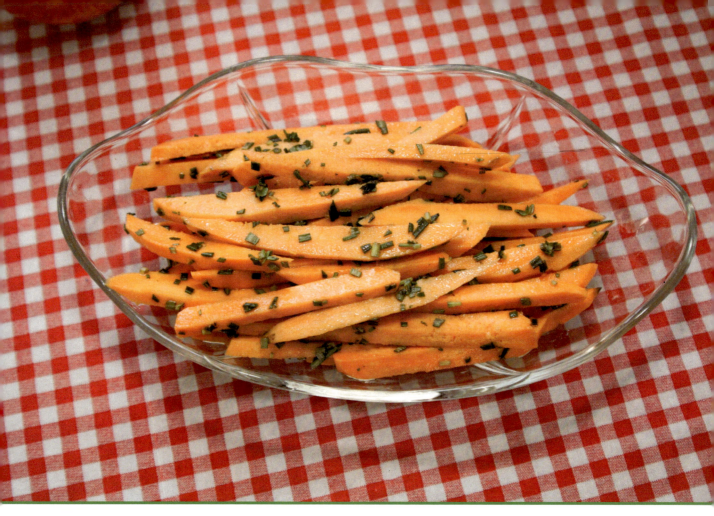

Spicy Jicama Fries

1 large jicama (2 pounds)
    (or, sweet potatoes)
1 T extra virgin olive oil
1 T paprika
1 t onion powder
1 t chili powder
½ t himalayan salt

Potassium

Monounsaturated Fat
Vitamin C
Sulphur
Capsaicin
Electrolytes

Blood

Skin
Immune System
Hair
Cardiovascular
Nerves

Peel and wash Jicama. Cut it into nearly equal thin strips. Take a large bowl and add all the ingredients - Jicama strips, olive oil, paprika, onion powder, chili powder and salt. Toss till you get a well blended mixture. Transfer into serving platters and enjoy. You can also serve these healthy Jicama fries after sprinkling with lime juice.

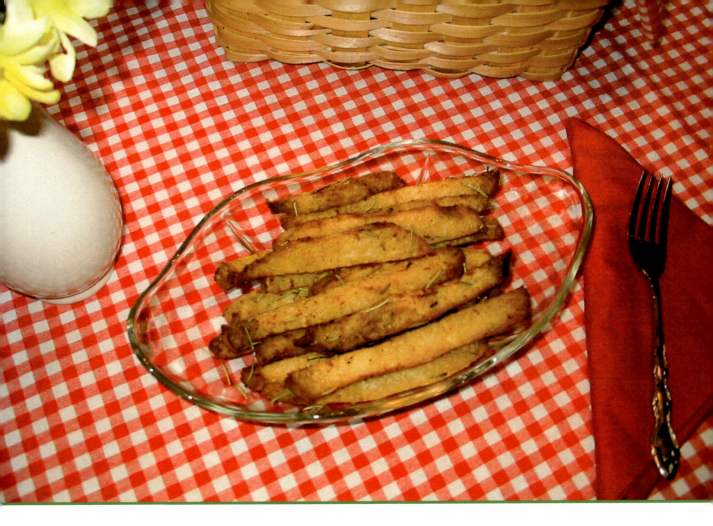

Savory Jicama Fries

1 large jicama (2 pounds)
    (or, sweet potatoes)
1 T extra virgin olive oil
1 T chopped rosemary
½ t himalayan salt

Potassium　　　　　　　　　Blood

Monounsaturated Fat　　　Skin
Choleric　　　　　　　　　　Antidepressant
Electrolytes　　　　　　　　Nerves

Peel and wash Jicama. Cut it into nearly equal thin strips. Take a large bowl and add all the ingredients Toss for even coating and serve.

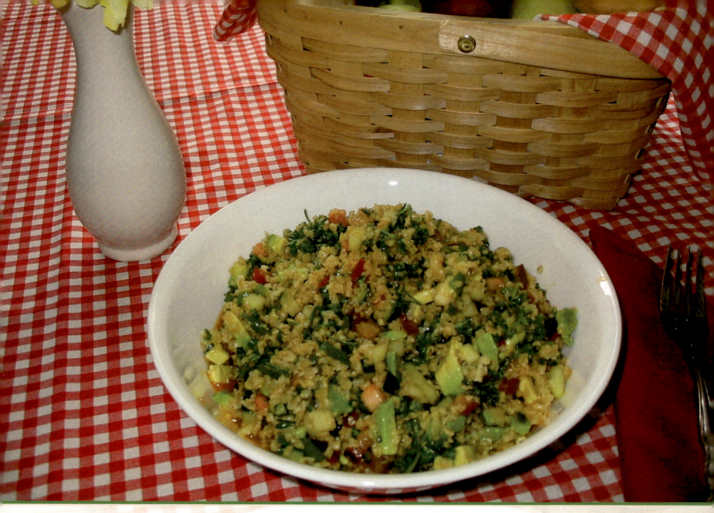

Tabouli

1 C bulger wheat, soaked overnight	**Ferulic Acid**	Anti Cancer
½ C parsley, finely chopped	**Vitamin C**	Immune System
½ C cucumber	**Silica**	Myofascial Layer
1 t himalayan salt	**Electrolytes**	Nerves
2 tomatoes	**Lycopene**	Anti Cancer
½ C scallions	**Sulphur**	Hair
¼ C lemon juice	**Vitamin C**	Immune System
1 clove garlic	**Allicin**	Antibiotic
1/3 C extra virgin olive oil	**Monounsaturated Fat**	Skin
1 avocado	**Carotenoid Lutein**	Eyes, Skin
1 t coriander	**Linoleic Acid**	Anti Arthritic
1 t mustard powder	**Selenium**	Cardiovascular
1 t paprika	**Vitamin C**	Immune System

Mix bulgar wheat, parsley, cucumber, salt tomatoes and scallions together in bowl and set aside. Blend together the lemon juice, garlic and olive oil. Pour over mixture in bowl. Cover and refrigerate for at least an hour so flavors can soften and blend.

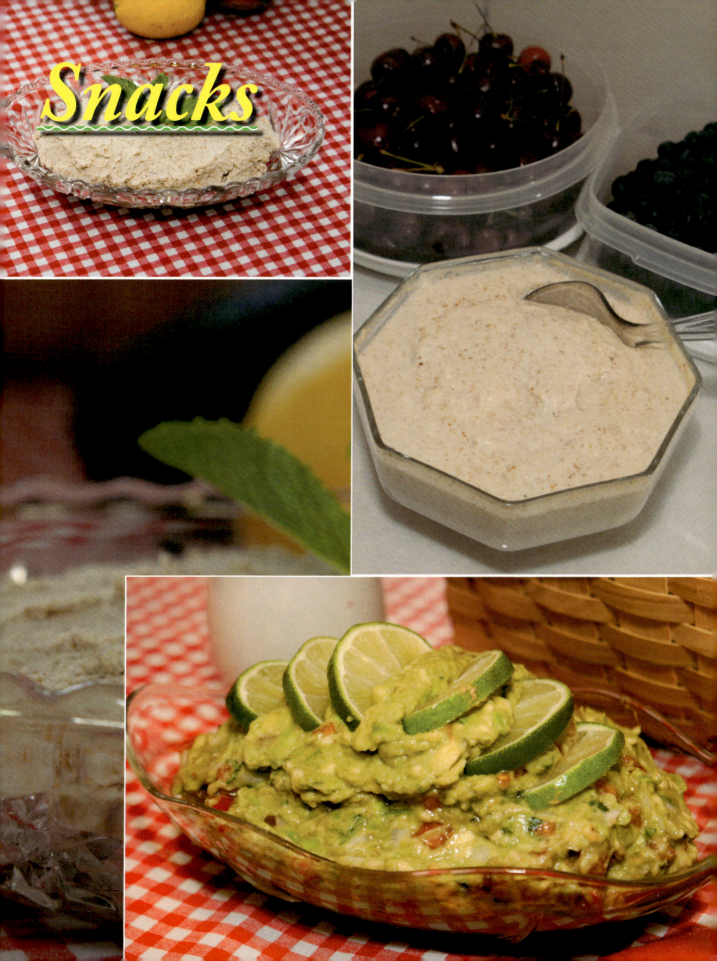
Snacks

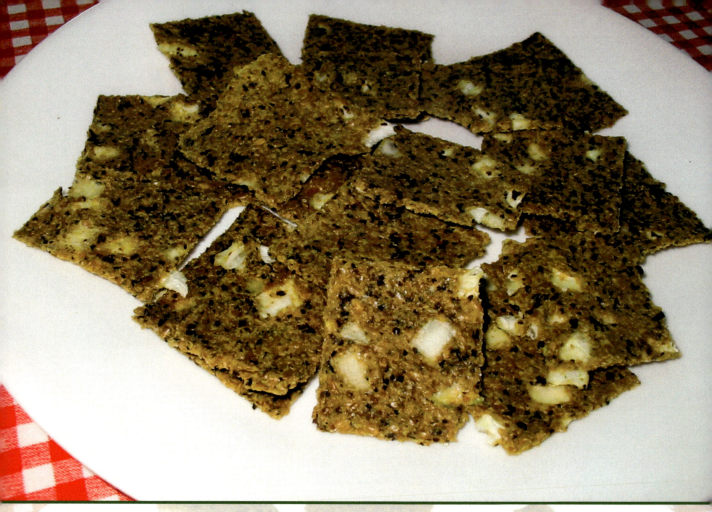

Flax Crackers

1 C flax seeds
1/8 C kelp flakes (or wakame)
2 C water

Essential Fatty Acids
Iodine
Oxygen

Hair
Thyroid
Cell Respiration

Let flax seeds soak for 30 minutes. Add kelp/wakame and spread onto the dehydrator tray. Dehydrate for 4 hours, flip, and dehydrate for another 4 hours or so until crispy.

Get creative! Make them sweet with cinnamon, raisins, and agave. Use the pulp from the almond milk and grind the flax seeds instead of leaving them whole, add a little agave and make more crackers or use for a pie crust.

Other ingredients to try include basil, garlic, onions, chili powder, chives, and celtic sea salt.

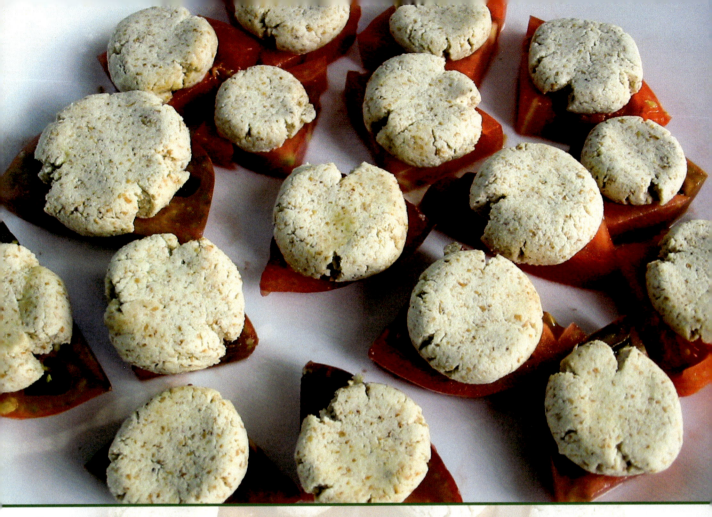

Savory Almond Ricotta Cheese

2 C almond pulp
1 clove garlic
1 T lemon juice
1 T miso
1 T nutritional yeast
1 T chopped onion
2 T tahini

Calcium — Bones
Allicin — Antibiotic
Vitamin C — Immune System
Amino Acids — Muscles
Lithium — Blood Pressure
Sulphur — Hair
Vitamin B3 — Positive Mood

Almond pulp is left over from making almond milk. Combine in food processor and puree.

RECIPES FOR LIVING – *Raw Food*

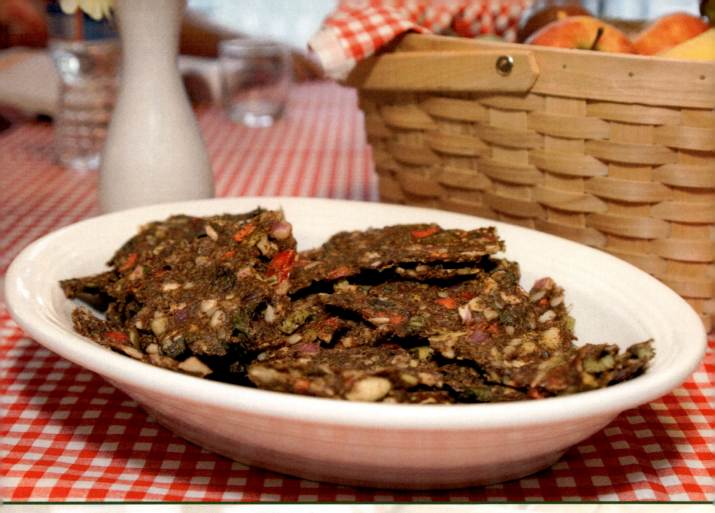

Brian's Famous Flax Crackers

1 C ground flax seeds (ground in coffee grinder)	**Essential Fatty Acids**	Hair
1 C water	**Oxygen**	Cell Respiration
½ C red onion, chopped fine	**Sulphur**	Hair
½ C tomato, chopped fine	**Lycopene**	Anti Cancer
½ C celery, chopped fine	**Sodium**	Stiff Joints
½ C basil, chopped fine	**Vitamin K**	Bones
¼ C sunflower seeds	**Vitamin E**	Cardiovascular
¼ C pumpkin seeds	**Zinc**	Prostate
¼ C coconut aminos	**Amino Acids**	Muscles
¼ C extra virgin olive oil	**Monounsaturated Fat**	Skin

Mix all ingredients in a bowl. Let sit for 15 minutes to thicken. Spread evenly on dehydrator trays with Teflex sheets. Dehydrate at 105 degrees F for 8-12 hours. Turn once and remove Teflex sheets mid-way through.

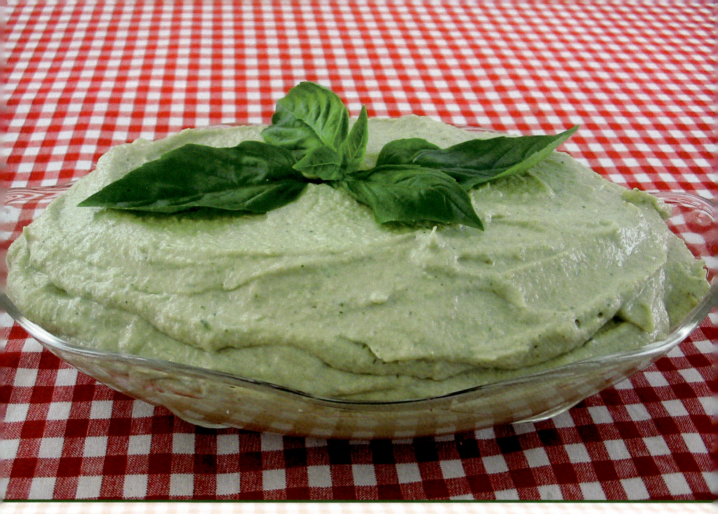

Zucchini Hummus

2 cloves garlic	**Allicin**	Antibiotic
¼ C lemon juice	**Vitamin C**	Immune System
1 zucchini, peeled & chopped	**Potassium**	Positive Mood
1/3 C water	**Oxygen**	Cell Respiration
2 C sunflower seeds	**Vitamin E**	Cardiovascular
1/3 C extra virgin olive oil	**Monounsaturated Fat**	Skin
½ C raw tahini	**Vitamin B3**	Positive Mood
2 t himalayan salt	**Electrolytes**	Nerves

In blender, mix the sunflower seeds until finely ground. Add all the rest of the ingredients and blend until well mixed and creamy.

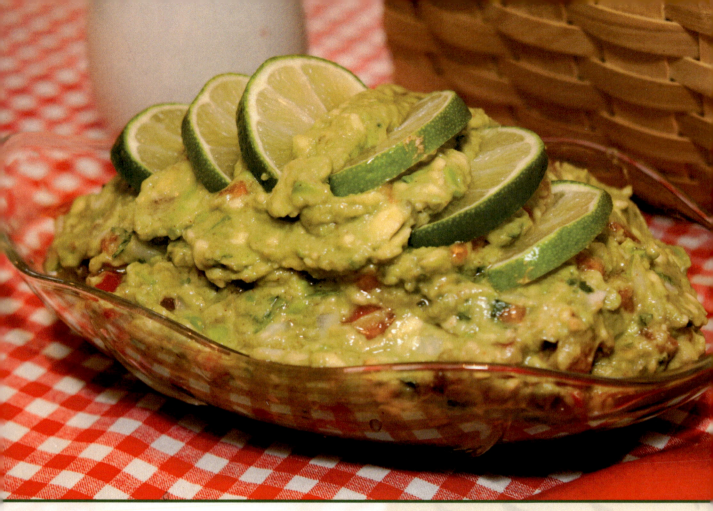

Guacamole

- 3 avocados
- 1 diced tomato
- ½ C diced red onion
- ½ C cilantro, chopped fine
- 1 clove garlic, diced fine
- 1 diced serrano pepper
- 1 juiced lime
- 1 t himalayan salt
- 1 t Bragg's Apple Cider Vinegar®
- ½ t ground cumin

Carotenoid Lutein	Eyes, Skin
Lycopene	Anti Cancer
Sulphur	Hair
Vitamin A	Skin
Allicin	Antibiotic
Capsaicin	Endorphins
Flavonoids	Skin
Electrolytes	Nerves
Vitamin B12	Positive Mood
Antioxidants	Anti Aging

In a large bowl place the scooped avocado pulp and lime juice, toss to coat. Drain, and reserve the lime juice, after all of the avocados have been coated. Using a potato masher add the salt and cumin and mash. Then, fold in the onions, tomatoes, cilantro, and garlic. Add 1 tablespoon of the reserved lime juice. Let sit at room temperature for 1 hour and then serve.

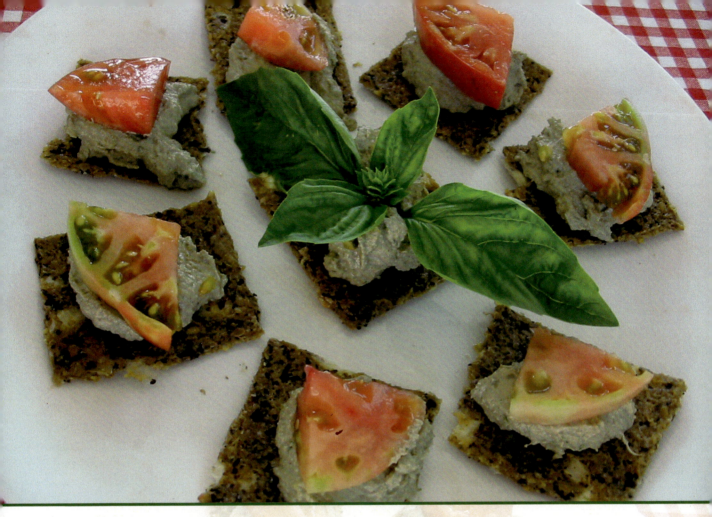

Walnut Hummus

3 C soaked raw walnuts
¼ C lemon juice
1 medium clove garlic
½ small onion
2 heaping T raw tahini
3 T extra virgin olive oil
1 t himalayan salt
1 t cayenne powder

Vitamin E	Brain
Vitamin C	Immune System
Allicin	Antibiotic
Sulphur	Hair
Vitamin B3	Positive Mood
Monounsaturated Fat	Skin
Electrolytes	Nerves
Capsaicin	Endorphins

Blend to pudding texture. If necessary, add a small amount of water to get the pudding consistency. The hummus will thicken after being refrigerated.

RECIPES FOR LIVING

Spicy Nacho Kale Chips

Ingredients	Nutrient	Benefit
1 bunch of curly kale (stems removed)	**Calcium**	Bones
½ C sprouted raw pumpkin seeds	**Zinc**	Prostate
½ C sprouted raw sunflower seeds	**Vitamin E**	Cardiovascular
2 cloves garlic	**Allicin**	Antibiotic
2 stalks celery	**Sodium**	Stiff Joints
1 tomato	**Lycopene**	Anti Cancer
4 stalks green onion	**Sulphur**	Hair
1 thumbnail-sized piece ginger	**Gingerols**	Digestion
1 juiced lemon	**Vitamin C**	Immune System
1 t cumin	**Antioxidants**	Anti Aging
2 t cayenne powder	**Capsaicin**	Endorphins
1 t himalayan salt	**Electrolytes**	Nerves
1 T raw agave	**Inulin**	Cardiovascular
2 T nutritional yeast	**Lithium**	Blood Pressure

Blend all ingredients except for kale in a blender. Place kale in a large bowl and pour in blender mix. Using your hands, massage thoroughly with love. Place kale evenly onto dehydrator trays one layer thick. Dehydrate at 105 degrees F for 12 hours.

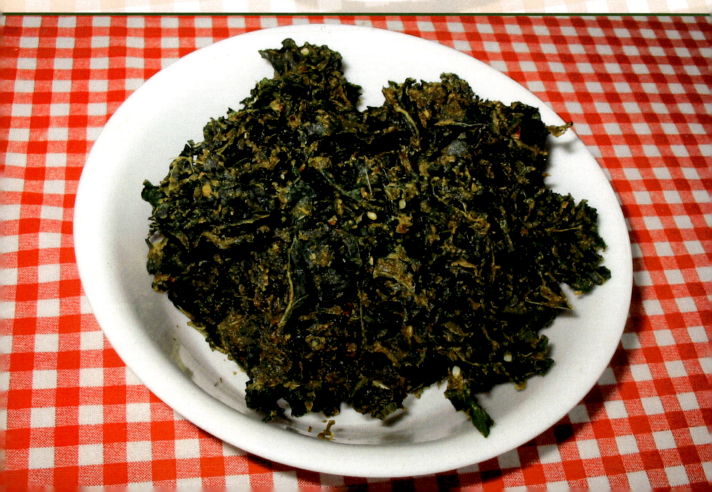

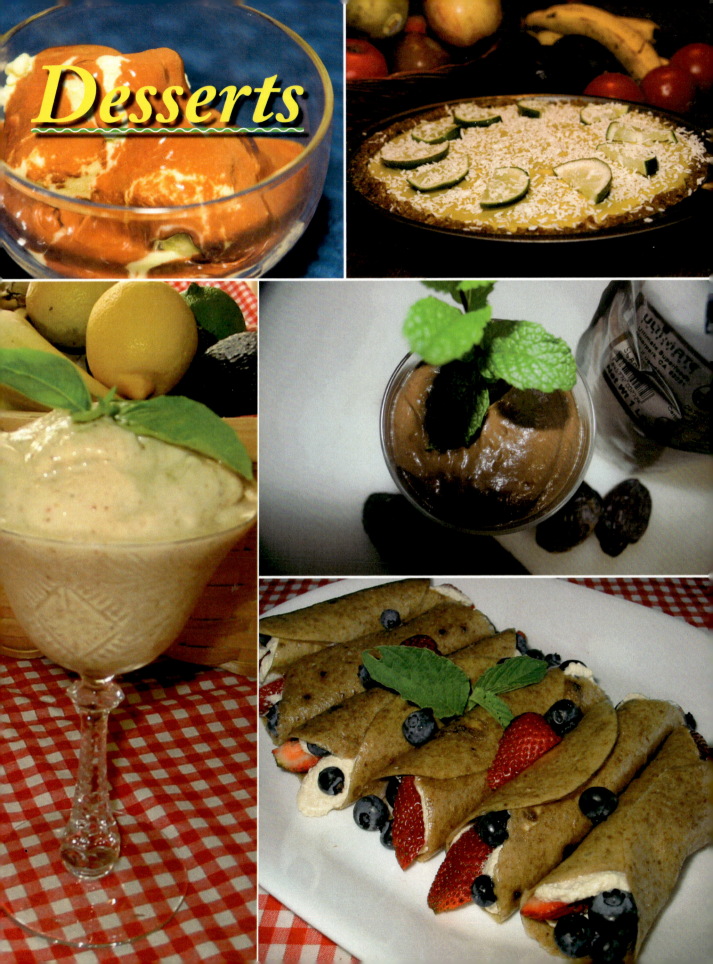

Desserts

RECIPES FOR LIVING

Cacao Power Balls

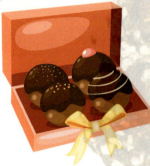
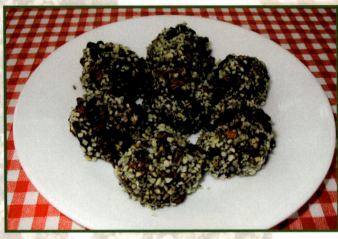

2 T agave nectar	**Inulin**	Cardiovascular
¼ C cacao nibs	**Magnesium**	Stress Relief
½ C cacao powder	**Magnesium**	Stress Relief
2 T coconut oil	**Lauric Acid**	Anti Aging
¼ C goji berries	**Antioxidants**	Anti Aging
¼ C hemp seeds	**Amino Acids**	Muscles
¼ C maca powder	**Testosterone**	Hormones

Put coconut oil in a bowl, start adding ingredients and mix. Mixture will condense and you can roll into balls. Roll balls in hemp seeds or cacao nibs. Yum!

Chocolate Macaroons

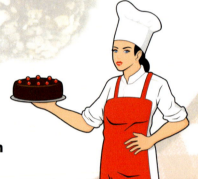

3 C dried coconut flakes	**Lauric Acid**	Immune System
1 ½ C cocoa powder	**Magnesium**	Stress Relief
1 C raw coconut nectar	**Vitamin C**	Immune System
½ C coconut oil	**Lauric Acid**	Anti Aging
1 T vanilla extract	**Aphrodisiac**	Need I Say More?
½ t sea salt	**Electrolyte**	Cell Communication

In a large bowl, combine all the ingredients and stir well to combine.

Using a small ice cream scoop or a big tablespoon, spoon rounds of the dough onto tray.

Garnish with pecans.
Place in freezer for 2 hours.

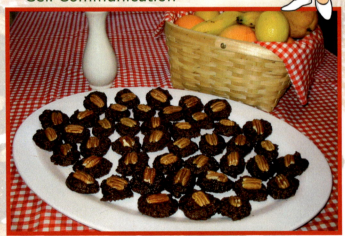

Raw Food - NATURAL VIBRANT HEALTH

NATURAL VIBRANT HEALTH – RAW FOOD

Chocolate Brownies

Brownie

1 C walnuts
1 C medjool dates
¼ C raw cacao

Vitamin E
Antioxidants
Magnesium

Brain
Anti Aging
Stress Relief

Icing

2 avocados
½ C agave nectar
¼ cup raw cacao
2 T coconut oil
1 T vanilla extract
1 dash himalayan salt
1 dash cinnamon

Carotenoid Lutein
Inulin
Magnesium
Antioxidant Lauric Acid
Aphrodisiac
Electrolytes
Manganese

Eyes, Skin
Cardiovascular
Stress Relief
Anti Aging
Need I Say More?
Nerves
Memory

Put brownie ingredients in a food processor and blend. Press into a small pan. Put all icing ingredients into Vitamix blender, and blend till smooth. Spread icing over brownies and pop in freezer to set for 1 hr. then cut into 12 sections. Put in snack sized baggies.

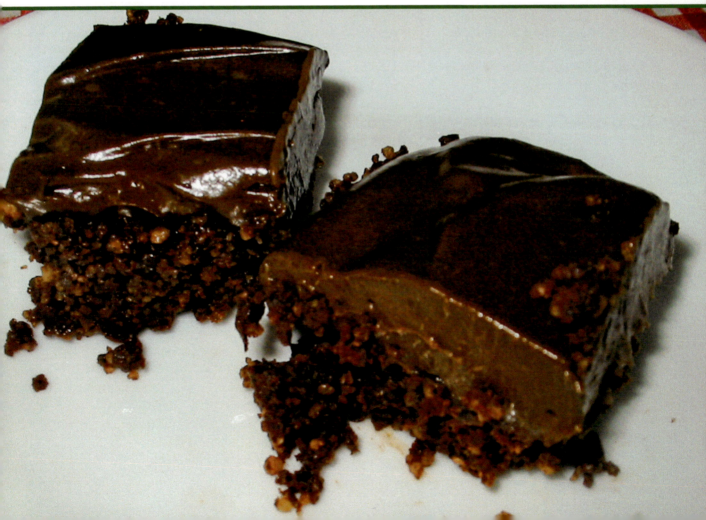

RECIPES FOR LIVING

Apple Pie

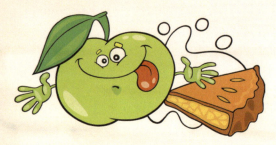
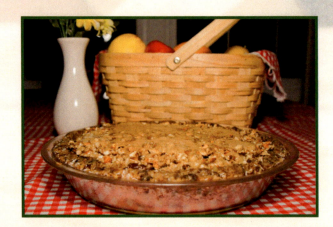

Crust

½ lb raw pecans	**Vitamin E**	Brains
1 C medjool dates	**Antioxidants**	Anti Aging
2 T shredded coconut	**Antioxidant Lauric Acid**	Anti Aging
1 t cinnamon	**Manganese**	Memory
2 pinches himalayan salt	**Electrolytes**	Nerves

Mix in food processor and then form into pie pan.

Filling

5 apples (peeled and cored)	**Antioxidants**	Anti Aging
1 C dates	**Antioxidants**	Anti Aging
¼ C raw agave	**Inulin**	Cardiovascular
2 T cinnamon	**Manganese**	Memory

Blend half of the apples with remaining ingredients. Pour half of apple mix into the pie crust. Finely slice remaining apples and put into the pie crust. Pour remaining apple mix on top.

Topping

½ C almonds	**Calcium**	Bones

Lightly blend almonds to make a crumbly topping and sprinkle on top of the pie.

Drizzle Garnish

¼ C raw agave	**Inulin**	Cardiovascular
2 T raw cacao powder	**Magnesium**	Stress Relief
2 T almond butter	**Calcium**	Bones

Blend. Drizzle on top to garnish.

Raw Food - NATURAL VIBRANT HEALTH

Brian's Famous Blueberry Cheesecake

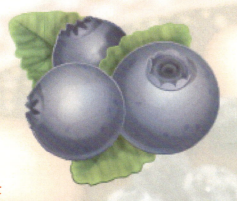
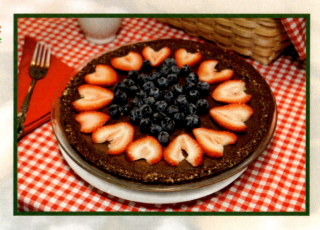

Crust

½ lb raw walnuts (soaked overnight)	**Vitamin E**	Brain
1 C medjool dates (soaked 20 minutes)	**Antioxidants**	Anti Aging
2 T shredded coconut (optional)	**Lauric Acid**	Anti Aging

Mix in food processor and then form into pie pan.

Filling

1 lb raw cashews (soaked 2 hours)	**Magnesium**	Stress Relief
½ C raw agave	**Inulin**	Cardiovascular
¾ C coconut oil	**Lauric Acid**	Anti Aging
½ C water	**Oxygen**	Cell Respiration
1 t vanilla extract	**Vanilloid**	Aphrodisiac
½ t himalayan salt	**Electrolytes**	Nerves
½ C blueberries	**Antioxidants**	Anti Aging

Blend and pour into pie crust.

Topping

¼ C raw agave	**Inulin**	Cardiovascular
½ C coconut oil	**Lauric Acid**	Anti Aging
½ C raw cacao powder	**Magnesium**	Stress Relief

Hand mix and pour on top.

Garnish with fresh strawberries and blueberries.

-- Bon appetite!

Recipes for Living

Key Lime Pie

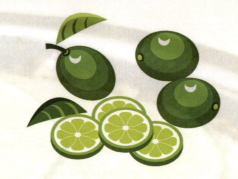

Crust

½ lb pecans
1 C medjool dates, soaked & drained

Vitamin E — Brain
Antioxidants — Anti Aging

Mix in food processor until it balls up. Sprinkle 2 Tbs. shredded coconut in a pie pan. Add crust ingredients and press evenly into the pie pan.

Filling Ingredients

2 small ripe avocados
1 banana
1 ¼ C juice from limes
½ C mango pieces
½ C agave nectar
1/3 C coconut oil
1 ½ t vanilla extract

Carotenoid Lutein — Eyes, Skin
Potassium — Blood
Flavonoids — Skin
Vitamin A — Eyes
Inulin — Cardiovascular
Lauric Acid — Immune System
Vanilloid — Aphrodisiac

Blend until smooth and fluid. Pour into pie pan and freeze about 4-6 hours or longer.

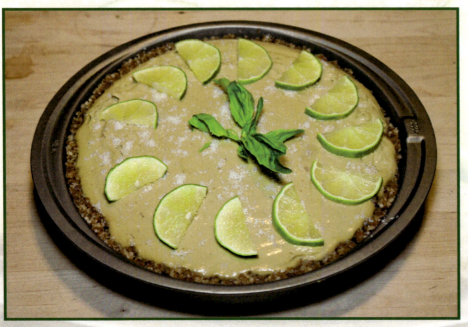

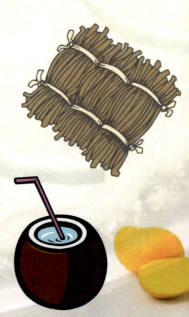

NATURAL VIBRANT HEALTH – RAW FOOD

Peach Pecan Cobbler

4 peaches
½ C dates
2 T lemon juice
2 T raw sesame seeds
1 t cinnamon
1 pinch sea salt
1 C chopped pecans

Phosphorous
Antioxidants
Phytonutrients
Essential Fatty Acids
Manganese
Electrolytes
Vitamin E

Skin
Anti Aging
Immune System
Cardiovascular
Memory
Nerves
Brain

Blend sesame seeds into a paste adding some of the reserved date water as necessary. When you have a paste add dates, lemon juice & sea salt. Add the necessary amount of reserved date water to create a thick caramel textured sauce. Cut peaches into slices and layer in a low casserole dish, sprinkle the cinnamon throughout. Cover the peaches with the date caramel sauce in your own artistic fashion. Sprinkle the pecans over the top

This step is optional. Place the casserole dish in a dehydrator for 45 minutes at 105°f.

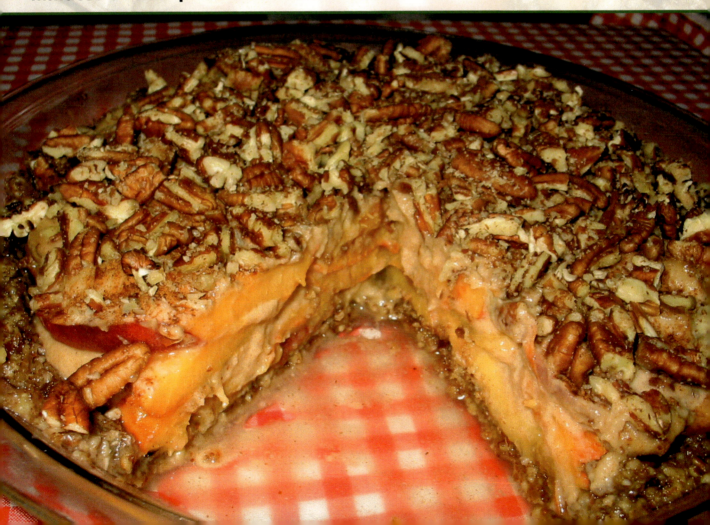

RECIPES FOR LIVING

Pumpkin Pie

Crust

½ C dates	**Antioxidants**	Anti Aging
2 C pecans	**Vitamin E**	Brain

The pecans should be soaked overnight and the dates soaked for 20 minutes. Combine in food processor and pulse until mixed evenly. Press into a glass pie plate.

Filling

½ C almond butter	**Calcium**	Bones
¼ t apple juice	**Antioxidants**	Anti Aging
¼ t cardamom	**Phytochemical Cineole**	Digestive System
2 t cinnamon	**Manganese**	Memory
½ t cloves	**Potassium**	Blood Pressure
1 C dates	**Antioxidants**	Anti Aging
1 t grated ginger root	**Gingerols**	Digestion
½ t nutmeg	**Myristicin**	Memory
2 C pumpkin meat	**Carotenes**	Antioxidant

The dates should be soaked for 20 min. Peel, seed and chop the pumpkin meat. Combine all ingredients in a food processor and puree. Spoon filling into crust and serve.

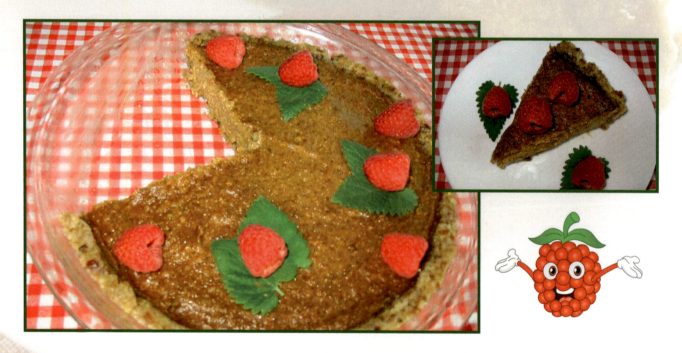

NATURAL VIBRANT HEALTH – RAW FOOD

Strawberry Crepes

Crepes

4 bananas
1 juiced lemon

Potassium
Phytonutrients

Blood Pressure
Immune System

Place bananas in food processor. Add lemon juice and process until liquid. Pour into 5" rounds. These should only be about 1/8" thick so spread mixture if necessary. Dehydrate overnight at 115. Do not over dry these. I start them just before I go to bed. You want them to be flexible. Makes 8 – 5" rounds.

Cashew Vanilla Cream

2 young thai coconuts (meat only)*
1 C cashews, soaked overnight
1 splash of Madagascar Vanilla®
1 T agave

Lauric Acid
Magnesium
Vanilloid
Inulin

Anti Aging
Stress Relief
Aphrodisiac
Cardiovascular

* Save the coconut water for smoothies, soups, or just drink it!

Place the cashews in high-speed blender. Blend on high speed. Add the coconut meat and vanilla. Process until well blended. Refrigerate to thicken if needed.

Assembly: Spoon the Cashew Vanilla Cream into half the crepe. Top with berries and add more cream. Fold over and experience joy!

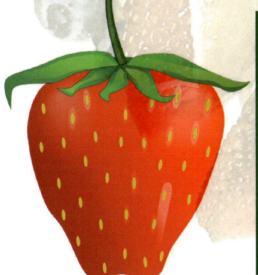
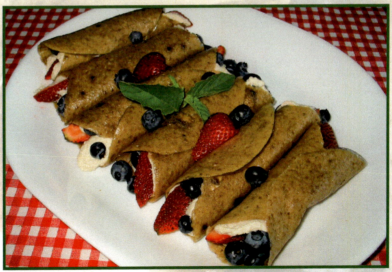

RECIPES FOR LIVING – *Raw Food* - 101

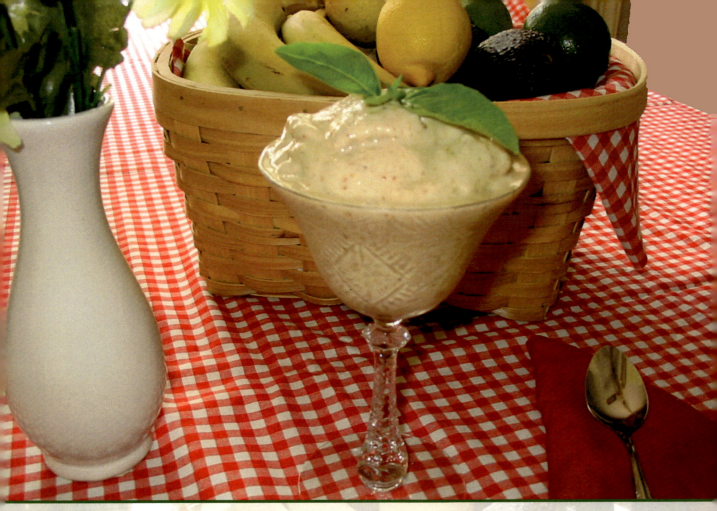

Ice Cream

8 medjool dates
1 C raw cashews
8 ice cubes
½ C water

Antioxidants
Magnesium
Oxygen
Oxygen

Anti Aging
Stress Relief
Cell Respiration
Cell Respiration

Blend! Unbelievably simple and delicious!

NATURAL VIBRANT HEALTH – RAW FOOD

Chocolate ~~Moose~~, Er... Mousse!

¾ C dates soaked
2 avocados
1 C almond milk
½ C almond butter
¾ C cacao powder
½ C agave

Antioxidants — Anti Aging
Carotenoid Lutein — Eyes, Skin
Calcium — Bones
Calcium — Bones
Magnesium — Stress Relief
Inulin — Cardiovascular

In a blender, combine all ingredients and blend or process until smooth. Refrigerate, then enjoy. You will not believe how good this is!

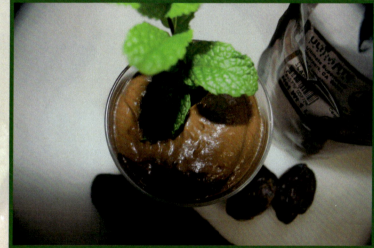

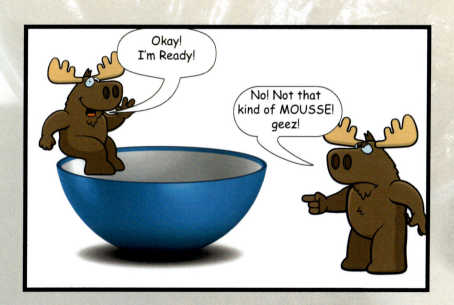

RECIPES FOR LIVING – *Raw Food* - 103

RECIPES FOR LIVING

Raw Food Studies

Eating nothing but raw, plant-based foods is such a radical idea to some people that they sometimes inquire about the existence of clinical research that support such a lifestyle. While there seems to be a plethora of scientific studies that validate the health benefits of vegetarianism or veganism, less well know is the preponderance of evidence that argue the even greater health benefits of eating raw food. Here are just a few notable examples of such research:

Pottinger's Cats

In 1932 Francis Pottinger, M.D. conducted a 10-year study on 900 cats to test the raw vs. cooked food diets. He divided the cats into two groups and fed the first group only raw foods and fed the second group the same exact same food only it was cooked.

The first group of cats fed raw food remained healthy, had good bone structure and density, were playful, were easy to handle, and they produced healthy kittens year after year with ease.

The second group of cats that were fed cooked food developed cancer, heart disease, arthritis, osteoporosis, glandular malfunctioning, kidney disease, sexual impotency, paralysis, skin diseases, allergies, pneumonia, difficulty in labor and severe irritability (making the cats difficult to handle.) The first generation of kittens born to the cooked food cats were ill or abnormal. The second generation were born either already diseased or dead.

The experiment had to be terminated early because by the third generation the mothers were sterile! The excrement from the cooked food cats was so toxic that the plants fertilized with it were stunted and weak; whereas the plants grown in soil fertilized by the excrement of the raw food cats grew normally.

Dr. Pottinger conducted similar tests on white mice. His results were identical to those in the cat experiment.

Enzyme Nutrition

Starting in the 1930's Dr. Edward Howell conducted 55 years of scientific research on humans on the subject of raw foods and enzyme depletion caused by eating cooked food over a lifetime. His groundbreaking studies revealed that enzymes are the catalysts for all biological processes and that life cannot exist without them. He also discovered that while raw, living foods are teaming with enzymes that cooking completely destroy them due to their sensitivity to heat. Enzymes within any given food make the digestion of that food possible. Eating cooked food not only denatures the food but also forces the body to steal metabolic enzymes in an attempt to digest the enzyme depleted food. Dr. Howell was able to make a direct correlation between eating enzyme depleted cooked food and the onset of chronic degenerative disease in humans. Dr. Howell's conclusion – *"many if not all, degenerative diseases that humans suffer and die from are caused by the excessive use of enzyme-deficient cooked and processed foods."*

Goldot

Lewis E. Cook, Jr. and Junko Yasui performed experiments comparing the effects of raw foods versus cooked foods in rats. The experiment involved three groups of rats.

The first group was fed a diet of only raw foods. They grew into completely healthy specimens and never suffered any diseases. They grew rapidly, never became fat, reproduced with vigor and enthusiasm, and produced healthy offspring. They were always playful and affectionate. Upon an age equivalent to 80 human years they were put to death and autopsied. All their organs, glands and tissues appeared in perfect condition without any signs of aging or degeneration.

The second group of rats were fed, from birth, diets of cooked foods. These rats became fat and were afflicted by the very same diseases afflicting present day society including: colds, fevers, pneumonia, poor eyesight, cataracts, heart disease, arthritis, cancer, etc. during the life-cycle of the second group, the rats exhibited vicious, nervous, and self-destructive behavior. They had to be separated to keep from killing each other. Their offspring were consistently ill and displayed the same behavioral characteristics as their parents. Most of the second group died prematurely from diseases or various epidemics which swept through the colony. Autopsies performed on this group revealed extensive degeneration in all the organs, glands, and tissues of their bodies.

The third group of rats were fed a diet identical to the second group until they reached the equivalent human age of 40 years. They displayed the same symptoms of ill-health and self-destructive behavior as the second group. At the end of this time period, the rats were placed on a strict water fast for several days. Then they were fed the raw diet of the first group. This diet was alternated with periods of fasting. Within one month their health and behavior patterns changed dramatically. They became affectionate, playful and never became ill. Autopsies performed after the human equivalent of 80 human years indicated this group had reversed its degenerative tissue damage.

Dr. Paul Kouchakoff

Dr. Paul Kouchakoff of the Institute of Clinical Chemistry in Lausanne Switzerland reported in 1930 that the white blood cell count goes up dramatically when eating cooked food indicating its toxic effect on the body. However, the chemical makeup of blood does not change when consuming raw food.

RECIPES FOR LIVING

Sir Robert McCarrison

Sir Robert McCarrison in India conducted a study where he fed monkeys their usual diet, but in cooked form. The previously healthy monkeys all developed severe intestinal problems. The autopsies reveled gastric and intestinal ulcers. Subsequent experiments on rats and the Hunza people (generally considered to be the healthiest population in the world), McCarrison concluded that a natural, raw food diet and healthy bodily activity is the best defense against degenerative diseases.

O. Stiner

O. Stiner in Switzerland conducted a study where he fed guinea pigs their usual diet, but in cooked form. His previously healthy animals succumbed to numerous diseases including: anemia, scurvy, goiter, dental carries, glandular degeneration and arthritis.

Heat & Pasteurization

"The Effect of Heat Treatment on the Nutritive Value of Milk for the Young Calf: The Effect of Ultra-High Temperature Treatment and of Pasteurization", British Medical Journal (Vol. 14, No. 10), 1960.

This study entailed feeding calves their mother's milk after it had been pasteurized. As a direct result of consuming this heat processed milk, 90% of the calves in the test died before reaching maturity.

Nutrition and Physical Disease

In the 1930's Dr. Weston A. Price, a dentist, traveled all over the world to study health and nutrition on primitive and isolated cultures. Repeatedly he found that natives whose diets consisted largely of whole, raw natural fruits and vegetables were free from those diseases common in civilized countries. They had healthy straight teeth and symmetrical dental arches. In contrast, natives of those same tribes and groups who moved to the cities and ate refined, cooked, packaged, processed and preserved "civilized" food, quickly degenerated. The teeth degenerated first. Second generation children had narrower facial bone structures, poorly formed dental arches and soft teeth that decayed rapidly.

And Much, Much More!

There are many other clinical studies that support the health benefits of eating raw food. For the sake of brevity the list is abbreviated here. There is also a plethora of anecdotal evidence of the power of raw foods. These are personal testimonies of people who have experienced increadible benefits of eating this way which has returned amazing results such as dramatic weight loss, reversal of health challenges, freedom from depression, improved mental clarity and other life-enhancing benefits.

Food Glossary

Here are details on some of the unusual ingredients used in our recipes some of which may be unfamiliar to you. Most of these items can be found in a hard-core health food store, may be carried by a very health-conscious nutritional consultant or are available on the internet.

Agave Nectar is a sweetener from the agave cactus plant which is native to the southwestern part of the United States and Mexico. It has a lower glycemic index compared to white sugar, maple syrup, honey, and high fructose corn syrup. Glycemic Index (GI) is the ranking of a food's immediate effect on blood sugar levels. There have been some health concerns recently regarding the use of agave nectar. You may want to consider using coconut nectar, coconut crystals or stevia for sweeteners – all of which have an even lower GI compared to agave nectar. Consumption of all sugars should be avoided by diabetics and those who are in the conquest of an illness.

Almond Butter is made from blending almonds to a paste. It is a healthier choice compared to peanut butter. Peanuts are easy targets for fungus because they are the only nuts that grow underground. Aflatoxin, a highly toxic mold, is commonly digested when consuming peanuts or any product made with peanuts. Almonds contain no aflatoxin. Almond butter is considered hypoallergenic, making it much easier for people with food allergies to eat. Almond butter also contains monounsaturated fats, a much healthier alternative to saturated fats. Monounsaturated fats reduce levels of cholesterol and decrease the risk of heart ailments. Almonds are an excellent source of calcium.

Anise is an herb used in many different ways. It is consumed after meals to help in the process of digestion. It is antimicrobial, has several compounds that are estrogenic, is used as an expectorant, and is used for sexual problems.

Ashwaganda is an herb from India known for improving blood flow and circulation to the limbs. Practitioners of Ayurvedic medicine claim that it can help increase libido.

Astragalus is an herbal supplement that comes from a type of bean or legume. It is best known for boosting the immune system. Astragalus is used widely in Chinese medicine for conditions such as the common cold, upper respiratory infections, fibromyalgia, diabetes, and heart disease.

Blue Green Algae is also known as Spirulina. An excellent variant of blue green algae is Aphanizomenon flos-aquae (AFA) from Klamath Lake in Oregon. Because of its' high protein (over 50%!), vitamin, and mineral content, blue green algae is considered a superfood. It is extremely nourishing. Blue green algae is a single cell organism that has not yet decided if it wants to be a plant or an animal. Because it is so low on the food chain it is elementary and foundational for restoring and repairing the body. Its' therapeutic effect is very powerful.

RECIPES FOR LIVING

Bragg's Apple Cider Vinegar® adds a tart flavor to recipes. It comes from the fermentation of apple juice and since it is raw, it contains beneficial living enzymes, Probiotics and B12. Once digested, it has an alkalizing effect on the body and draws out toxins. Bragg's Apple Cider Vinegar is good for relieving the pain of gout, rheumatoid, and osteoarthritis.

Bragg's Liquid Aminos® like soy sauce adds a salty flavor to recipes. Since it has no added table salt, MSG, or preservatives it is a healthier alternative to soy sauce. Bragg's Liquid Aminos® is made from certified non-GMO soybeans. It is a good source of amino acids which are the building blocks of protein.

Cacao Powder is made from raw cacao beans that have been dried, powdered, and minimally processed. It is an excellent source of magnesium, phytochemicals, polyphenols, and antioxidents. The Theobromine in cacao is known for cognitive enhancement and mood. Other chemicals that naturally occur in cacao include MAI inhibitors which diminish appetite, PEA which is similar to what the brain releases when we are in love, and anadamide which is the "bliss" chemical (the same chemical released when we are very happy). Raw cacao is also good for the brain and the heart.

Cacao Nibs are also made from cacao beans that have been chopped into small bits. They have all the same health benefits of cacao powder. Cacao nibs add a dimension of texture to recipes.

Celtic Sea Salt is usually found on the coastal areas of France. Its light grey, almost light purple color comes from the clay found in the salt flats. The salt is collected by hand using traditional Celtic methods. This type of salt replenishes electrolytes, contains 82 trace elements, and trace minerals. It is a raw product that has not been cooked or devitalized. It is a good source of naturally occurring iodine. Unlike table salt, Celtic Sea Salt® has no chemical additives, has not been bleached, diluted with anti-caking agents, and has not had all the beneficial minerals and trace elements removed. Salt helps bring out the flavor in foods. In order to maintain the proper sodium/potassium ratio in the body, salt should be used sparingly.

Coconut Aminos adds a salty flavor to recipes. Unlike soy sauce, Coconut Aminos® is raw and contains no added table salt, MSG, or preservatives. It is a good source of amino acids which are the building blocks of protein. Coconut Aminos® is an excellent choice for people who wish to avoid soy.

Coconut Crystals is a raw, low glycemic (GI of only 35) sugar alternative made from coconut tree sap. It is dried and resembles the consistency of brown sugar. Coconut Crystals® is an abundant source of vitamins, minerals, and amino acids.

Raw Food - NATURAL VIBRANT HEALTH

Coconut Flakes are made from dried and shredded coconut meat. Unlike other saturated fats which, upon being consumed are stored in fat cells, the medium chain fatty acids in coconuts are absorbed directly by the liver. This means they produce energy much faster, raising the body's metabolism which helps burn more calories, contributing to weight loss. The lauric acid and monolaurin, found in coconut flakes have antibacterial, antiviral properties and boost the immune system.

Coconut Nectar like Coconut Crystals is a raw, low glycemic (GI of only 35) sugar alternative made from coconut tree sap. It is in the syrup form and resembles the consistency of molasses. Coconut Nectar® is an abundant source of vitamins, minerals, and amino acids.

Coconut Oil is extracted from pressed coconut meat. The medium chain fatty acids in coconut oil is not like other saturated fats as they are absorbed directly by the liver, not stored in fat cells. This means they produce energy much faster, raising the body's metabolism. This helps burn more calories, contributing to weight loss. The lauric acid and monolaurin, found in coconut oil have antibacterial, antiviral properties and boost the immune system. Coconut oil is a very versatile product and can be eaten and used externally on the skin.

Coconut Water is the juice in the interior of young coconut The liquid is clear, sweet, and sterile and composed of vitamins, minerals, electrolytes, enzymes, amino acids, cytokine, phyto-hormones, and sugars. Coconut water is a very refreshing drink to beat thirst by replenishing hydration levels in the body. The water has the highest source of electrolyes known to man. Some research studies suggest that cytokinins (e.g., kinetin and trans-zeatin) in coconut water showed significant anti-ageing, anti-carcinogenic, and anti-thrombotic effects.

Cordyceps is a mushroom that parasitically grows out of the heads of rare Tibetan insects at altitudes of over 18,000 feet. It is normally available in a dried, powdered form or in capsules. It is adaptogenic (meaning it helps you manage stress) and is known as an aphrodisiac. Cordyceps is known to increase energy, endurance, stamina, oxygen capacity, lung function, lung capacity, immune system, and improves sexual function. It also battles weakness and fatigue and is very popular with endurance atheletes of all types. Today, most cordyceps are grown on barley and other less disgusting nutrient sources.

Dulse is a red sea vegetable and has a mildly spicy and salty sea flavor. It is dried and chopped into flakes. Dulse is an excellent source of vitamins, minerals, and trace elements. It is an especially good source of iodine which is good for the thyroid.

Fenugreek is an herb that is commonly found growing in the Mediterranean region of the world. In Ayurvedic and Chinease medicine it has also been used for arthritis, asthma, bronchitis, improve digestion, maintain a healthy metabolism, increase libido and male potency, skin problems, treat sore throat, and cure acid reflux. Fenugreek contains phytoestrogens and is used for breast enlagement and to increase milk production in breastfeeding mothers.

RECIPES FOR LIVING

First Cold Pressed Organic Olive Oil is extracted from the first pressing of olives. It is a good source of monounsaturated fats which is good for the skin and heart. "Cold-pressed" organic means the oil is extracted without using heat or chemicals to assist in the extraction process. "First cold-pressed" means the olives are run through the press one time (instead of multiple times as is otherwise the case) for better flavor and nutrient value. "First cold-pressed" and "extra virgin" mean the same thing.

Flax Oil is extracted from pressed flax seeds. It is an excellent source of proteins, vitamins, minerals and balanced essential fatty acids including omega 3, 6 and 9. These essential fatty acids have a short shelf life and flax oil should be kept refrigerated.

Flax Seeds are an excellent source of proteins, vitamins, minerals and balanced essential fatty acids including omega 3, 6 and 9. The seeds are also an excellent source of fiber. The whole seeds are too difficult to digest and should be ground to extract all the nutritional benefits. Because of its' highly perishable nature, flax seeds should be ground just prior to consumption and not ahead of time.

Ginkgo Bilabo is an herbal supplement extracted from the leaves of huge, stately ginkgo trees which can be found growing all over the United States. Because ginkgo improves blood flow and oxygenation to the brain and limbs it is used for Alzheimer's and other age-related conditions. It improves alertness, memory, the ability to concentrate, and improving mood.

Ginseng is an herbal supplement extracted from the root of the Ginseng plant. Popular varieties are found in both America and Asia. Many Asians consider ginseng as the herbal fountain of youth and certain rare varieties fetch over $100,000 per plant! It is a warming herb increasing motion of the blood and circulation to the limbs. It tones the skin and muscles, boosts the immune system and increases sexual energy. Athletes use Ginseng to increase strength and endurance.

Goji Berries are a bright orange-red berry that comes from a shrub that's native to Tibet and parts of China. Goji is considered a superfood because it is one of the world's most nutrient-dense foods. They are so loaded with vitamins, minerals, antioxidants, and phytonutrients that they are truly in a league of their own. In fact, of all the natural substances that have been researched, Goji berries have been found to contain more beta carotene than any other food! For example, Goji berries have ten times the antioxidants of blueberries, fifty times the beta carotene of carrots and more iron than a steak! In traditional Chinese medicine, it is believed that Goji berries increase sexual fluids, fertility, longevity, and boost the immune system.

Green Powder is a whole food supplement made from dried and powdered green plants. Our favorite type of green powder is VitaMineral Green® by HealthForce Nutritionals. It has an impressive array of whole-food sourced vitamins, minerals, herbs, superfoods, sea vegetables, energenic mushrooms, beneficial algeas, digestive enzymes, Probiotics, and trace elements. For example, the ingredients include Nettle leaf, Shavegrass (horsetail), Alfalfa leaf juice, Dandelion leaf juice, Barley grass, Oat grass juice, Wheatgrass, American basil, Holy basil, Moringa leaf, Yacon leaf, Nopal cactus, Chickweed, Ginger root, Broccoli juice, Kale juice, Spinach juice, Carob pod, Amla berry, Spirulina, Chorella, Icelandic kelp, Dulse, Nori, Alaria, Bladderwrack, Protease, Amylase, Lipase, Cellulose, Bromelain, Papin, Alpha-galactosidase, and Shilajit.

He Shou Wu is sometimes called "Fo Ti". It is an ancient Chinese herb with a reputation for anti-aging, boosting vitality, virility, and longevity. He Shou Wu is a powerful kidney, liver and sex tonic. He Shou Wu is said to improve the cardiovascular system, enhances immune functions, slows the degeneration of glands, increases antioxidant activity, and reduces the accumulation of lipid peroxidation. This herb is also said to increase essence and blood - a combination of attributes that increase fertility in women and sperm in men. He Shou Wu has even been known to restore natural hair color in some people. "He" is the family name, "Shou" means head, "Wu" means black. The literal translation of He Shou Wu would mean "Mr. He with a Head of Black Hair."

Hemp Seeds are rich in protein, fiber, vitamins, minerals, antioxidants, and phytonutrients. They contain all the essential amino acids and essential fatty acids good for muscle and tissue development necessary to maintain and build healthy human life. Hemps seeds are an excellent and balanced source of omega 3, 6, and 9 essential fatty acids.

Himalayan Salt is mined from caves high in the Himalayan mountains. It replenishes electrolytes, contains many trace elements, and trace minerals. It is a raw product that has not been cooked or devitalized. It is a good source of naturally occurring iodine. Unlike table salt, Himalayan salt has no chemical additives, has not been bleached, diluted with anti-caking agents, and has not had all the beneficial minerals and trace elements removed. Salt helps bring out the flavor in foods. In order to maintain the proper sodium/potassium ratio in the body, salt should be used sparingly.

Horsetail is an herbal supplement that is a good source of silicon which plays an important role in repairing skin, bone, cartilage, arteries, and connective tissue. The active components from horsetail have antimicrobial, antiseptic, anti-inflammatory effects and they preserve eyesight and stimulate blood flow. It is also used for digestive problems, bronchitis and pneumonia. Horsetail is a good source of selenium and silicon which both help promote circulation to the scalp which helps maintain healthy hair. It is excellent when used for osteoporosis.

RECIPES FOR LIVING

Jicama is a legume native to tropical and subtropical Central America. It is high in potassium and carbohydrates in the form of dietary fiber. It is composed of 86-90% water; it contains only trace amounts of protein and lipids. Its sweet flavor comes from the oligofructose inulin (also called fructo-oligosaccharide), which the human body does not metabolize; this makes the root an ideal sweet snack for diabetics and dieters.

Kelp Flakes is a green sea vegetable and has a mildly spicy and salty sea flavor. It is dried and sold in sheets, chopped into flakes, or as a powder. Kelp is an excellent source of vitamins, minerals, and trace elements. It is an especially good source of iodine which is good for thyroid health.

Maca is native to the high Andes mountains of Peru. It only grows at an altitude over 14,000 feet, in areas of intense sunlight, strong winds and below freezing temperatures – where no other crops can survive. The root of the plant is used in a dried and powdered form. Its nutrient profile is impressive as it is rich in protein, essential minerals, especially selenium, calcium, magnesium, and iron. Maca also contains essential fatty acids including linolenic acid, palmitic acid, and oleic acids, as well as polysaccharides. Maca is an adaptogen which helps you deal with stress and is an athletic performance enhancer. It is an aphrodisiac and it's reported beneficial effects for sexual function is partly due to its high concentration of proteins and vital nutrients. Maca also contains unique sterols which are similar to many of the hormones in your body.

Medjool Dates are considered to be the diamond of dates and are prized for their large size, extraordinary sweetness and chewy texture. Dates are rich in fiber as well as several vitamins and minerals including calcium, sulphur, iron, potassium, phosphorous, manganese, copper and magnesium. They have abundant antioxidants which neutralize the effects of free radicals. Dates help in fighting constipation and boost sexual function. Medjools were once highly prized and exclusively reserved for members of the royal Morrocan family.

Mesquite Powder adds a sweet, nutty taste to your recipes similar to carob with carmel undertones. The bean pods of the mesquite are dried and ground into flour. Mesquite is a leguminous plant found in the southwestern United States and Mexico. It is good for balancing blood sugar levels and is a good source of fiber. Mesquite also contains lysine (an amino acid), as well as notable quantities of digestible protein, calcium, magnesium, potassium, iron and zinc.

Miso is a traditional Japanese food produced by fermenting rice, barley and/or soybeans. It adds a salty dimension to your recipes. Miso is high in protein and rich in vitamins and minerals.

Nama Shoyu is a Japanese soy sauce that is not pasteurized. It is produced from roughly equal quantities of soybean and wheat. It is a good source of amino acids which are the building blocks of protein.

Nori Sheets is the Japanese name for various edible seaweed or "sea vegetables". It is made by shredding and rack-drying seaweed in a process that resembles paper-making. Japan, Korea, and China currently are the major producers. Nori is an excellent source of vitamins, minerals, and trace elements. It is an especially good source of iodine which is good for thyroid health.

Nutritional Yeast is a deactivated yeast that is used as a nutritional supplement and as a condiment. Nutritional yeast has a nutty, cheesy, creamy flavor which makes it popular as an ingredient in cheese substitutes. It is an excellent source of protein and vitamins, especially the B-complex vitamins. It is also naturally low in fat and sodium. It comes in the form of flakes, or as a yellow powder similar in texture to cornmeal, and can be found in the bulk section of most hard-core health food stores.

Rhodiola is an adaptogen which means it increases the body's ability to deal with stress of all kinds. It is known to increase energy, endurance, stamina, mood, promote better sleep, mental clarity, mental performance, and sexual performance. It is also known to reduce stress and anxiety.

Stevia is a South American plant which is used in the place of sugar. It is a no-glycemic sweetner with a glycemic index (GI) of 0.

Stinging Nettle is an herb that commonly grows along riverbanks. It has the flavor of spinach and is rich in vitamins A, C, iron, potassium, manganese, and calcium. It is used medicinally for arthritis, gout, baldness, memory loss, allergies, hives, respiratory troubles, coughs, runny nose, chest congestion, and asthma. There is a process called "urtication" which literally means intentionally flogging oneself with stinging nettles! This act of deliberately applying stinging nettles to the skin provokes inflammation and is done in order to increases blood flow due to the release of histamines. This provides relief from the pain of rheumatism.

SunWarrior Protein Powder® is a sprouted, fermented whole grain brown rice. At 83% protein, Sunwarrior Protein Powder® has the highest (non soy) raw whole grain sprouted vegan protein on the market. Naturally rich in vitamins and minerals, Sunwarrior Protein contains high amounts of antioxidants tocopherols, and tocotrienols and other essential nutrients such as thiamin, riboflavin, niacin, phosphorous, iron and potassium.

Tahini is a paste made from ground sesame seeds. It is a major ingredient in hummus and other Middle Eastern dishes. Sesame seeds are a very good source of manganese, copper, calcium, magnesium, iron, phosphorus, vitamin B1, zinc and dietary fiber. In addition to these important nutrients, sesame seeds contain two unique substances: sesamin and sesamolin. Both of these substances belong to a group of special beneficial fibers called lignans, and have been shown to have a cholesterol-lowering effect in humans, and to prevent high blood pressure and increase vitamin E supplies in animals. Sesamin has also been found to protect the liver from oxidative damage.

RECIPES FOR LIVING

Teeccino® is an herbal coffee substitute. It is available in several different flavors. The ingredients include things like carob, barley, chicory root, dates, figs, and almonds. Unlike coffee, Teeccino is non-acidic which is desirable for persons with gastrointestinal conditions like acid reflux and IBS. Teeccino contains the prebiotic, inulin which is a soluble fiber from chicory root that supports a healthy population of beneficial digestive flora necessary for good digestive health. Teeccino provides two heart-healthy nutrients, potassium, an electrolyte mineral, and soluble fiber. Potassium helps prevent strokes and high blood pressure. Soluble fiber lowers total cholesterol.

Wakame is a red sea vegetable and has a mildly spicy and salty sea flavor. It is dried and chopped into flakes. Wakame is an excellent source of vitamins, minerals, and trace elements. it's a good source of other minerals including magnesium, iodine, calcium, and iron. It's also high in vitamins A, C, E, and K as well as folate and riboflavin. It's also a good source of lignin. Wakame is an especially good source of iodine which is good for the thyroid.

Yohimbie is an herbal supplement from the bark of an evergreen tree in West Africa. This herb is claimed to work as an aphrodisiac and may also help with depression and high blood pressure.

Young Thai Coconuts are imported from Thailand and are in their early stages of growth when they are the most nutritious. We use the water and the meat in recipes. The water has the highest source of electrolytes known to man. Unlike other saturated fats which, upon being consumed are stored in fat cells, the medium chain fatty acids in coconuts are absorbed directly by the liver. This means they produce energy much faster, raising the body's metabolism which helps burn more calories, contributing to weight loss. The lauric acid and monolaurin, found in coconut have antibacterial, antiviral properties and boost the immune system. There is no cholesterol in young Thai coconuts.

Index

A

absorption 60
acid 60, 64
acid forming 60
acidosis 64
acne 10
ADA 59
adrenaline 65
agave 86, 92, 94, 95, 96, 97, 98, 101, 103
Alexander the Great 12
alkaline 64
alkaline-ash 60
allergies 10, 104
allicin 50, 71, 34, 87, 89, 90, 91, 92
almond butter 35, 53, 59, 96, 100, 103
almond milk 29, 59, 86, 87, 103
almond pulp 87
almonds 35, 52, 59, 96
American Association of Drugless Practitioners 9
amino acids 26, 87, 88, 94
anemia 26, 106
animal 13, 65
animal protein 60
anise 47
anti aging 27, 90, 92, 95, 96, 97, 98, 99, 100, 101, 102, 103
anti arthritic 57, 52, 57, 66
antibacterial 71, 83
antibiotic 50, 65, 87, 89, 90, 91, 92
anti cancer 50, 88, 90, 92
antidepressant 70, 75
anti-histimine 47
antioxidant Allicin 75
antioxidant Carvacrol 69
antioxidant Lauric Acid 51, 95, 96
antioxidants 27, 47, 53, 90, 92, 94, 95, 96, 97, 98, 99, 100, 102, 103
aphrodisiac 29, 94, 95, 97, 98, 101
apple 28, 74, 96
apple cider vinegar 64
apple juice 100
apple pie 96
arthritis 39, 46, 104, 105, 106
arugula 47
Ashwaganda 47
Astragalus 26
autopsies 105, 106
avocado 62, 90, 95, 98, 103

B

backaches 10
banana 26, 29, 27, 28, 31, 32, 34, 35, 37, 39, 98, 101
basil 31, 52, 56, 62, 67, 69, 71, 75, 77, 78, 81, 86, 88
beautiful skin 25
beef 63
beet 43
beet tops 33
bell pepper 57
beta carotene 17, 43, 50, 67, 71
Bio-Individual Health Evaluation Education 9
blood 32, 27, 28, 29, 31, 52, 56, 62, 67, 69, 71, 75, 77, 78, 82, 83, 98
blood glucose 9
blood pressure 26, 32, 33, 56, 57, 66, 68, 69, 70, 75, 87, 92, 100, 101
bloodstream 41
blood sugar 54, 79
blueberries 31, 34, 97
blueberry cheesecake 97
blue-green algae 27
blue smoothie 33

bok choy 59
bone 47
bone health 50
bones 29, 87, 88, 92, 96, 100, 103
Bragg's Apple Cider Vinegar® 90
Bragg's Liquid Aminos® 81
brain 35, 47, 91, 95, 96, 97, 98, 99, 100
brain fog 10
brazil nuts 66
bread 74
Brian Clement 9
Brian Hetrich 10
Brian's Famous Blueberry Cheesecake 97
Brian's Famous Flax Crackers 88
bright eyes 25
broccoli 59, 62
bromelain 39
brownie 95
B.S. in Biology and Psychology 9
bulger wheat 84
buns 81
burgers 81
burritos 66
butternut squash 53

C

cacao 95
cacao nibs 94
cacao powder 27, 35, 94, 96, 97, 103
Cacao Power Balls 94
calcium 29, 46, 47, 50, 52, 56, 57, 61, 64, 66, 67, 87, 92, 96, 100, 103
calories 60
cancer 13, 105
capsaicin 28, 50, 90, 91, 92
carbohydrates 41
cardamom 100

cardiovascular 28, 52, 54, 56, 61, 66, 76, 84, 88, 89, 92, 96, 97, 98, 99, 101, 103
cardiovascular disease 64
carnivore 65
carotenes 53, 100
carotenoid lutein 26, 67, 90, 98, 103
carotenoids 54, 43
carrot 41, 43, 33 70
cashew 39, 66, 69, 97, 101, 102
Cashew Sour Cream 66
Cashew Vanilla Cream 101
casserole dish 99
catalyst 13
cataracts 105
cats 104
cattle 65
Cauliflower Rice 62, 68
Cauliflower Sprout Salad 62
cayenne powder 28, 52, 67, 91, 92
celery 26, 88, 92
cell communication 54, 94
cell respiration 32, 86, 88, 89, 97, 102
celtic sea salt 86
Center for Educational Outreach and Innovation 9
champagne mango 26, 76
champion 17
Cheesecake 97
"Cheeze" Sauce Topping 70
Cheezy Cauliflower Casserole 70
chelation 57
chemical reaction 13
cherries 28
Cherry-Fire Smoothie 28
chicken 63
Chili 76
chili powder 66, 86
chives 86
chlorogenic acid 57, 55
Chocolate Brownies 95
Chocolate Macaroons 94

Chocolate Mousse 103
choleric 70
cholesterol 60
chronic ailments 10
chronic degenerative disease 104
cilantro 46, 90
cineole 66
cineole acid 57
cinnamon 29, 86, 95, 96, 99, 100
cleansing 9
clearing your mind 41
clear thinking 25
clinical research 104
cloves 100
cobbler 99
coconut 56, 96, 97
coconut aminos 52, 88
coconut flakes 94
coconut meat 54
coconut milk 54
coconut nectar 94
coconut oil 27, 94, 95, 97, 98
coconut water 26, 61, 67, 46, 50
colds 105
collagen 62
collard 72
collard greens 26, 59
Cometa Wellness Center 9
commercial food distribution 13
convection oven 13
cook 14
cooked food 14, 104, 105
cooking 13, 27
cooking process 64
copper 70
cordyceps 26
coriander 57
cow's milk 59
Crepes 101
crushed red pepper 75
crust 96, 97, 98, 100
cubes 102
cucumber 29
cultures 106

cumin 57, 90, 92
cuminaldehyde 57
curcumin 51

D

D3 serum 59
daily calcium requirement 60
dairy 59, 60, 65
dark leafy greens 65, 29, 13, 12
dates 3, 41, 95, 96, 97, 98, 99, 100, 102, 103
David Wolfe 74, 44
degeneration 105
degenerative diseases 106
dehydrator 13, 16, 86, 88, 92, 99
dental carries 106
dentist 106
depression 106
Desserts 93
diabetes 10
diet 9
digestion 13, 57, 77, 92, 100
digestive 14, 35
digestive enzymes 64
digestive system 100
digestive tract 72
dijon mustard 72
dill 64
disease 8
Doctor of Naturopathy 41
Doctor of Naturopathy in Original Medicine 77
Dolmas 62
Dr. Edward Howell 104
Dressing 3
Drinks & Juices 77
drizzle garnish 96
Dr. Paul Kouchakoff 105
Dr. Pottinger 104
Dr. Weston A. Price 106

E

Electrolytes 14, 26, 41, 89, 90, 91, 92, 94, 95, 96, 97, 99

elephants 65
endorphins 46, 90, 91, 92
Entrees 63
environmental pollution 65
enzyme nutrition 104
enzymes 13, 14, 33
epidemics 105
essential fatty acids 41, 56, 86, 88, 99
excalibur 17
excess mucus 64
excess weight 11
exercise 10
extra virgin olive oil 50, 88, 89, 91
eye 26, 50, 90, 98, 103

F

fasting 41
fat 60
fenugreek 47
fermented foods 9
fertility 47
Ferulic Acid 84
fevers 105
fiber 13
filling 96, 100
filling engredients 98
fish 63
flavonoids 66, 90, 98
Flax Crackers 86, 88
flax seeds 86, 88
folate 32, 74
food processor 13, 16, 87, 95, 98, 100
fountain of youth 25
free radicals 34
fruit 12, 106
Fruit Chard Smoothie 17

G

garlic 50, 51, 52, 55, 56, 57, 66, 69, 71, 72, 75, 76, 78, 81, 84, 86, 87, 89, 90, 91, 92

garnish 76
ginger 43, 44, 46, 50, 51, 53, 55, 56, 71, 79, 92, 100
gingerols 43, 46, 50, 51, 53, 55, 56, 71, 79, 92, 100
ginkgo bilabo 47
ginseng 47
giraffes 65
glands 105
glandular degeneration 106
glandular malfunctioning 104
glowing complexion 41
glutamine 63
glutathione 62
glycation 13
goiter 106
goji berries 27, 47, 94
golden flax seeds 74
Goldot 105
good health 12
gorillas 65
gourmet 12
grape leaves 77
grape tomatoes 76
green apple 33
green juices 41
green onion 92
green powder 26
green power 17
green smoothies 25
Green Star 17
Guacamole 66, 90
guinea pigs 106

H

habanero pepper 46
hair 27, 50, 82, 84, 86, 87, 88, 90, 91, 92
headaches 10
healing diseases 41
healing herbs 9
health and wellness 11
health challenges 11
health education lectures 11

healthy children 9
healthy meal planning 11
heart 26, 53, 71
heart disease 13, 104, 105
heat & pasteurization 106
heat sensitive 13
hemp seeds 94
herbivore 65
herophiles 12
high blood pressure 10
high cholesterol 10
high raw 10
high-speed blender 15
himalayan salt 31, 79, 81, 89, 90, 91, 92, 95, 96, 97
Holistic Health Counselor 9
honey 71
hormones 27, 60, 65
horses 65
horsetail 47
ho shu wu 47
Howell 104
humans 13
Hummus 89, 91
hunza people 106
hydration 41

I

Ice Cream 102
ice cubes 34, 79, 39, 44
icing 95
immune strength 71
immune system 27, 87, 89, 91, 92, 94, 98, 99, 101
immunity 9
improved mental clarity 106
increased energy 25, 41
India 106
ingredients 20
  fresh 20
  local 22
  organic 21
  plant-based 22
  raw 20

ripe 20
whole 21
Institute for Integrative Nutrition 9
Institute of Clinical Chemistry 105
Institute of Medicine 59
International Institute of Original Medicine 11
intestinal ulcers 106
intestines 43
inulin 35, 92, 94, 96, 97, 98, 101, 103
iodine 77, 86
IOM 59
iron 26
isolated cultures 106

J

Jake 6
jalapeno pepper 67, 81
jicama 82, 83
joints 43, 44, 46
juicer 17
julienne slicer 19
Junko Yasui 105

K

kale 26, 39, 44, 59, 61, 92
Kale Chips 92
Karma Fest 9
kelp flakes 86
Kendell Reichart 8
Kendell's Famous Raw Burritos 66
Kendell's Green Smoothie 26
Ketchup 81
Key Lime Pie 98
kidney 41
kidney disease 104
kitchen tools 15
kittens 104
Kombucha 45

L

labor 104
lasagna 69
lauric acid 27, 94, 97, 98, 101
Lausanne Switzerland 105
leaky gut syndrome 64
lemon 44, 12, 92, 101
lemon juice 51, 87, 89, 91, 99
lettuce 65
Lewis E. Cook, Jr. 105
libido 70
life energy 65
life-enhancing benefits 106
lime 90, 98
lime juice 66
linoleic acid 57
lithium 56, 87, 92
liver 46
living food nutrition 9
living foods 12, 14
local produce vs. conventional produce 9
low energy 10
Lutherville, MD 9
lycopene 50, 88, 90, 92
lysine 63

M

macadamia nuts 51, 69, 72
maca powder 27, 37, 94
Macaroons 94
Madagascar Vanilla® 101
magnesium 27, 60, 94, 95, 96, 97, 101, 102, 103
mandolin 19, 69
manganese 29, 95, 96, 99, 100
mango 26, 34, 69, 98
marinara 69, 67, 81
meat 65
medjool dates 35, 95, 96, 97, 98, 102
memory 29, 27, 35, 37, 39, 95, 96, 99, 100
mental clarity 11
metabolic 13
metabolic enzymes 14
microwave 13
minerals 13, 26, 52, 55, 56
miso 50, 87
mixing bowl 76
Mocha Chocolate Milkshake 35
molecules 63
monkeys 106
monosaturated fat 75
monoterpenes 72
monounsaturated fat 50, 51, 88, 89, 91
mucus 64
mung bean sprouts 50
muscle 26, 63, 81, 87, 88
muscle tissue 50
mushroom 55
mustard 72
mustard greens 59
mustard powder 84
myofascial 26, 84
myristicin 29, 100

N

nama shoyu 66, 81
natural killer cells 27
naturopath 10
nerves 27, 51, 53, 54, 61, 66, 67, 68, 69, 70, 72, 75, 76, 78, 79, 82, 83, 84, 89, 90, 91, 92, 95, 96, 97, 99
nettles 60
niacin 50, 77
noodles 69, 71, 78
nutmeg 29, 53, 100
nut milk bag 18
nutrient 41, 60, 63, 65
nutritional constituents 11
nutritional consultant 9
nutritional yeast 56, 57, 66, 68, 69, 70, 75, 87, 92
Nutrition and Physical Disease 106
nuts 59

O

okra 59
olives 62, 75
Omega-3 17
Omega-3 Fatty Acids 74
Omega Institute for Holistic Studies 9
one on one session testing 9
onion 51, 56, 57, 66, 67, 69, 75, 78, 81, 87, 91, 92
onion powder 82
onions 86
orange juice 71
oregano 69
organic gardening 9
organs 105
osteoporosis 13, 104
O. Stiner 106
overweight 10
oxygen 32, 86, 88, 89, 97, 102

P

Pad Thai 71
paprika 82, 84
paralysis 104
parasites 65
parsley 44
pasta 78
pasteurized 106
paté 81
peach 38, 65, 99
Peach Pecan Cobbler 99
pecans 66, 96, 98, 99, 100
pepper 50
pesto 69
phosphorous 38, 60, 99
physician 12
phytochemical cineole 100
phytoestrogens 47
phytonutrients 44, 41, 99, 101
pickle 72
pie 98
pie pan 98
pine 69

pineapple 39
Pizza 74
plant 13, 64
plant-based diet 10
plant-based foods 59, 104
plunger 16
pneumonia 104, 105
poor eyesight 105
poor vision 10
pork 63
portabella mushrooms 81
positive mood 50, 87, 89, 90, 91
potassium 26, 60, 63, 64, 65, 89, 98, 100, 101
potato masher 90
potlucks 11
Pottinger's Cats 104
prebiotic 35
processed 13
Professional Credentials 9
Professional Training Program 9
proline 63
prostate 62, 88, 92
protein 13, 14, 27
protein powder 26
pumpkin meat 100
Pumpkin Pie 100
pumpkin seeds 88, 92
puree 81, 87, 100

R

rabbit 65
raisins 86
raspberry 45
raspberry zinger 45
rats 105
raw agave 35
raw chocolate parties 9, 11
raw food 9, 12, 13, 14, 62, 106
raw food cooking classes 11
raw food diet 10
raw foodists 63
raw food kitchen 15
Raw Foods and Healing Herbs 9

Raw Food Studies 104
red bell pepper 57, 67
red onion 62, 75, 76, 88, 90
red pepper 69
respiration 70
respiratory 41, 67
rheumatic 66, 69
rhinoceros 65
rhodiola 47
ricotta 69
Ricotta Cheese 87
rosemary 70

S

SAD 10, 12, 14, 17
sage 68
salad 62
saliva 9
sauce 71
Savory Almond Ricotta Cheese 87
Savory Jicama Fries 83
scallion 55
scallions 52, 43, 44
SCOBY 45
scurvy 106
sea salt 66, 64, 86, 94, 99
Sedona, Arizona 3
seeds 59, 72
selenium 55, 12, 14
serrano pepper 90
sesame oil 56
sesame seeds 59, 99
severe irritability 104
sexual desire 47
sexual energy 47
sexual impotency, 104
sexual performance 47
shallots 50
shiny hair 25
shitake mushroom 50, 55
Sides 63
silica 26, 46, 60, 72, 77
Sir Robert McCarrison 106
skin 38, 88, 89, 90, 91, 98, 99,

103
skin diseases 104
sleep 10, 77
smoothies 25, 60
sodium 26, 34, 39, 88, 92
Soup 49
soy sauce 81
spaghetti 78
spatula 81
Spicy Jicama Fries 82
Spicy Nacho Kale Chips 92
spinach 26, 27
spiralizer 18
spirooli 18, 78
spring onion 50, 76
sprouting 9
sprouting jars 18
sprouts 59
Standard American Diet 10
Standardized Measurements 23
   ¼ Teaspoon 23
   1/8 Teaspoon 23
   1/16 Teaspoon 23
   4 Ounces 23
   8 Ounces 23
   12 Ounces 23
   big handful 23
   bunch 23
   C 23
   Cup 23
   dash 23
   handful 23
   pinch 23
   Q 23
   Quart 23
   splash 23
   t 23
   T 23
   Tablespoon 23
   Teaspoon 23
sterile 104
steroids 65
stiff joints 26, 88, 92
stinging nettle 47

stove 13
strawberries 32, 97
Strawberry Crepes 101
strengthened immune system 41
stress 34
stress reduction 72
stress relief 66, 95, 96, 97, 101, 102, 103
strong bones 60
stronger bones 41
Stuffed Bell Peppers 67
sugar 45
sugar addiction 9
Sulphur 50, 67, 78, 87, 88, 90, 91, 92
sun 65
sunbathing 60
sundried tomato 57, 69
sunflower seeds 67, 88, 89, 92
sunlight 41, 60
Sun Warrior Protein Powder 26
superfood parties 9
superfoods 9
sweet potato 54, 79
Sweet Potato Casserole 79
swiss chard 26
Switzerland 106

T

Tabouli 84
taco meat 66
tahini 59, 87, 89, 91
tamper 16
tea 60
Teachers College at Columbia University 9
Teeccino® 35
teflex sheets 74, 88
testosterone 27, 57, 94
thai coconut 56
The American Dairy Association 59
thyme 67, 75, 76
thymol 67
thyroid 77, 86

tissue development 26
tissues 105
tomato 50, 69, 88, 90, 92
tomato sauce 75
topping 71, 96
toxic 13, 65, 105
tryptophan 63
tuna wraps 72
turmeric 29
turnip greens 59

U

ulcers 106
Ultimate Smoothie 36
University of Maryland 9
unnatural foods 13
urine 9

V

vanilla 101
vanilla bean 35
vanilla extract 29, 35, 94, 95, 97, 98
Vanilloid 29, 42, 97, 98, 101
vegan 10
veganism 104
vegetable 12, 41, 106
vegetarian 10
vegetarianism 104
Veggie Miso Soup 50
Very Berry Smoothie 32
vibrant health 12, 44
vitamin A 26, 53, 62, 90, 98
vitamin B3 87, 89, 91
vitamin B12 90
vitamin C 28, 41, 87, 89, 91, 92, 94
vitamin D 60
vitamin E 35, 88, 89, 92, 95, 96, 97, 98, 99, 100
vitamin K 31, 88
vitamin P 46
vitamins 13
vitamin U 62

Vitamix 16, 95

W

wakame 86
Walnut Hummus 91
walnuts 35, 91, 95, 97
water 32, 86, 88, 89, 97, 102
water fast 105
weak bones 60
weight bearing exercises 60
weight loss 9, 106
weight management 11
Weston A. Price 106
wheatgrass 17
white blood cell count 105
wooden mallet 79
world hunger 65

Y

yohimbe 47
young thai coconuts 101

Z

zinc 62, 88, 92
zucchini 50, 69, 71, 78, 89
Zucchini Hummus 89

Be sure to visit these fine websites for great life changing information!

http://www.LivingFoodNetwork.Org
http://www.NaturalVibrantHealth.Net
http://www.GetMyHealthBack.Org